KEYGUIDE TO INFORMATION SOURCES IN

Paramedical Sciences

KEYGUIDE TO INFORMATION SOURCES IN

Paramedical Sciences

Edited by John Hewlett

MANSELL

LONDON AND NEW YORK

First published 1990 by
Mansell Publishing Limited, *A Cassell Imprint*
Villiers House, 41/47 Strand, London WC2N 5JE, England
125 East 23rd Street, Suite 300, New York 10010, U.S.A.

British Library Cataloguing in Publication Data
Keyguide to information sources in paramedical sciences.
  1. Medicine. Information sources
  I. Hewlett, John
  610.7

  ISBN 0-7201-2057-8

Library of Congress Cataloging-in-Publication Data
Keyguide to information sources in paramedical sciences / edited by
  John F. Hewlett.
     p.   cm.
  Includes bibliographical references.
  ISBN 0-7201-2057-8
  1. Medical literature. 2. Medicine—Bibliography. I. Hewlett,
John F.
  [DNLM: 1. Health Occupations—bibliography. 2. Health
Occupations—directories. 3. Information Services—directories.
ZW 21.5 K44]
R118.6.K49 1990
610—dc20
DNLM/DLC
for Library of Congress
                                            90-5863
                                              CIP

This book has been printed and bound in Great Britain
by Biddles Ltd., Guildford and King's Lynn.

Contents

PART II Bibliographical Listing of Sources of Information

PART III List of Selected Organizations

Foreword

During the past fifty years there has been a continuing exponential growth in the literature of medicine and health. The amount of available information on health has long since expanded beyond the capability of any one person to master it all. Indeed, in the early 1960s the vast accumulation of biomedical research information threatened to break down the American system for managing its scientific knowledge base. In response, the information profession has expanded to include librarians, information officers, brokers, documentalists and archivists. These people and others have together created a significant array of information tools – from directories, catalogues and bibliographies to complex automated databases – and the field of medical informatics has emerged.

Such developments have accompanied the emergence of the concept of the health care team, where professionals from various health-related disciplines contribute their skills to patient care. Information is no longer isolated or confined within specific professions but is available to be shared by different types of practitioner. Some of the paramedical professions have had a limited literature, which has reflected both the size of the profession and also its gradual development from being largely a body of practical skills to one that embraces a sounder theoretical base. Barely fifty years ago entry to some paramedical professions included a mere six to nine months of training where today a full graduate education is required spanning three or four years.

As a student of chiropody at the London Foot Hospital many years ago I can recall the limited library resources available at that time. Subsequently, on changing professions to medical librarianship I became aware of the considerable literature resources that are now available. The paramedical professions are poised for an exciting future where improved professional recognition is linked to a much stronger foundation of theory.

It is within this context that the present *Keyguide to information sources in paramedical sciences* has been compiled. The expertise of these authors has produced an informative and valuable guide to the sources of information available to the paramedical professions. Inevitably the use of this book will influence the training of professionals in their various disciplines. Both tutors and students can be guided to the wealth of information resources available and this must contribute significantly to the academic basis of the professions. But additionally the guiding to sources of information needed for professional practice and patient care will help to draw theory and practice together, while emphasizing the concept of the health care team.

Within each paramedical profession the body of specific literature is still not large and in some fields authoritative textbooks are still relatively rare. The periodicals literature is expanding rapidly, although it is also sometimes of uneven quality. A more significant problem is that this literature is often poorly indexed and suffers from incomplete coverage in the principal indexes and databases. The general picture that emerges is one where the paramedical literature is growing in stature but is not comprehensively available in National Health Service or university libraries, nor is it comprehensively accessible through the secondary indexes and abstracts.

In these circumstances this volume should prove to be a significant contribution to the health professions. It brings together much valuable information on the paramedical professions that is not easily available elsewhere. It should be of particular value to the libraries of paramedical educational establishments and could act as a stimulus to the development of the literature of those disciplines. It will also be of special value to National Health Service and university medical libraries where a multi-disciplinary approach is taken to support the work of health care teams.

The communication of professional knowledge through the literature is vital to the continuing development of all professions. This volume may become a significant milestone in the development of the paramedical professions, in the UK and elsewhere, and will be an important contribution to practice, research and education in these fields.

R. B. Tabor
Regional Librarian
Wessex Regional Health Authority

Preface

Paramedical or allied health professionals are usually considered to be those groups of health care workers who are not doctors or nurses, but who have a part to play in the diagnosis or cure of disease, the rehabilitation of the patient or the maintenance of his or her health. They include a wide range of staff groups, all of whom have a need for information for updating, for clinical and management decision-making, for education and for research.

This volume covers the information sources for six groups of allied health workers who treat patients directly and have their own defined literatures. They are chiropodists, dietitians, occupational therapists, physiotherapists, radiographers (both diagnostic and therapeutic) and speech therapists. The terms 'paramedical' and 'allied health' are used throughout this book to refer to these groups together.

The need for such a book became apparent when the editor was researching the information needs of paramedical staff in Haringey Health Authority. There had been little research on the subject, and little written to inform the paramedical personnel or the staff who supplied their library and information requirements. It is hoped that this book will help to fill this need.

The Contributors

Linda V. Castleton, TDCR(T), *Principal, South East Thames Regional Radiotherapy Education Centre, Lambeth Wing, St Thomas's Hospital, Lambeth Palace Road, London SE1 7EH, England.*

John Hewlett, MSc, ALA, *Regional Librarian, North East Thames Regional Library Service, North Middlesex Hospital, Sterling Way, London N18 1QX, England.*

Karen Hyland, SRD, *District Dietitian, Islington Health Authority, Whittington Hospital, Highgate Hill, London N19 5NF, England.*

Cathy Hyland, SRD, *District Dietitian, Haringey Health Authority, North Middlesex Hospital, Sterling Way, London N18 1QX, England.*

Mary Lovegrove, TDCR(R), DMU, *Senior Tutor (Radiography), Normanby College, School of Radiography, King's College Hospital, Denmark Hill, London SW5 9RS, England.*

Margie Mellis, MA, ALA, *Librarian, Grampian School of Occupational Therapy, Woolmanhill, Aberdeen AB9 1GS, Scotland.*

Pat Munro, BA, ALA, *Librarian, National Hospitals College for Speech Sciences, Chandler House, 2 Wakefield Street, London WC1N 1PG, England.*

Dave Roberts, BA, *Medical Information Service, British Library Document Supply Centre, Boston Spa, near Wetherby, West Yorkshire LS23 7BQ, England.*

Erica South, ALA, *Librarian, School of Chiropody, London Foot Hospital, 33 Fitzroy Square, London W1P 6AY, England.*

Graham Walton, MA, BSc, FETC, ALA, *Faculty Librarian (Social Sciences), Newcastle upon Tyne Polytechnic, Ellison Place, Newcastle upon Tyne NE1 8ST, England.*

PART I

Overview of Paramedical Sciences and Their Literature

1 Information and the Paramedical Professions

John Hewlett

DEFINITIONS

The paramedical professions are described in *Dorland's Illustrated medical dictionary* [128]* as those that are 'adjunctive to the practice of medicine in the maintenance or restoration of health and normal functioning'. Other dictionaries give more general definitions: *Mosby's Medical and nursing dictionary* [135] describes paramedical personnel as 'health-care workers other than physicians, dentists, podiatrists and nurses'; Miller and Keane [134] state that paramedical services include physiotherapy, occupational therapy, speech therapy, etc., and social work.

Only the *Wiley International dictionary of medicine and biology* [142] states that 'the specific range of application of "paramedical" varies from country to country'. In the USA the paramedical professions are usually known as allied health professions, and Brandon and Hill [18] state that they encompass 'as many as 200 health related professions and occupations'. In South Africa paramedical personnel are known as ancillary workers.

HISTORY IN THE UK

In order to regulate the paramedical professions in the UK, the British Medical Association (BMA) devised a licensing system which resulted in 1936 in the Board

---

* Numbers in square brackets are cross-references to items in the bibliography (Part II) or the list of organizations (Part III).

of Registration of Medical Auxiliaries (BRMA). Those in auxiliary occupations were permitted to work only under medical direction, and had to follow BMA requirements for their training. Larkin[20] has written further about the period leading up to 1960, with particular reference to the history in the United Kingdom of ophthalmic opticians, chiropodists, physiotherapists and radiographers.

Employment within the UK National Health Service (NHS) in paramedical fields was first restricted to professionally qualified staff by the NHS (Medical Auxiliaries) Regulations of 1954,[14] which followed the recommendations of the Reports of the Committees on Medical Auxiliaries, chaired by Cope.[24]

As paramedical staff looked for more independence and desired to get away from the label 'auxiliary', negotiations with the Ministry of Health led to the Professions Supplementary to Medicine Act of 1960,[15] which brought into existence the Council for the Professions Supplementary to Medicine (CPSM). The Council provides seven of the paramedical professions with a structure for professionalism – a means of statutory professional registration and a disciplinary body. These seven professions are chiropody, dietetics, medical laboratory technology, occupational therapy, orthoptics, physiotherapy and radiography (both diagnostic and therapeutic).

Each profession has a Statutory Registration Board operating as a separate autonomous body. Each is responsible for: identification and registration of the professionally competent (and for issuing a list of those registered to practise); approval of qualifications, examinations, training courses and schools; and enforcement of professional standards and discipline. The roles of the CPSM and the Boards are outlined further by Donald[12] and by a briefing in the *British Medical Journal*.[4] The CPSM also issues an annual report on its work.[9]

Speech therapists were considered by the Committees on Medical Auxiliaries, but later excluded themselves on the grounds that they are a free-standing profession in their own right, with as much relation to education as to medicine.

LIBRARY AND INFORMATION NEEDS

Information is needed and libraries are used by health care professionals for four main purposes: education, either basic or post-basic; clinical decision-making and updating; management; and research.

Roy Tabor was one of the first NHS librarians to consider user needs and information use. His DHSS/OSTI research project in 1971–73[29] aimed: to define the various categories of users in the health sciences; to determine the levels of information required; to establish the purposes for which the information was required; to investigate patterns of communication of information; and to distinguish the various sources of information available. Tabor concluded that information handling for the NHS was a national problem, with time and money being spent on local solutions that were often uncoordinated and incompatible.

He recommended 'the economic channelling of resources into an effective network which would benefit all categories of staff in the NHS'.

In 1982, Brember and Leggate[3] discussed user needs in health care, relating needs to libraries and particularly to NHS libraries. They referred to the professional diversity and hierarchies in the NHS, and to library provision, which has been traditionally separate for three main user groups – doctors, learner nurses and managers. 'Very often, minority groups are served by none of these.'

Recent work on user needs in health care has often been related to library use rather than to a broader information use. A seminar on library needs of the paramedical professions was reported briefly by Clark.[8] The seminar emphasized the lack of services available to this group, and stood in contrast with three similar seminars on libraries for medical staff, nursing staff and NHS managers. Clark stressed the need for access to libraries, the provision of current awareness services, abstracting and indexing services and a supply of bench books; she also stated the need for research-based literature (now growing rapidly in some disciplines) and for user education in library and information use at basic student level.

Proposals from a Joint Working Party of the Department of Health and Social Security (DHSS) and the NHS Regional Librarians' Group (RLG)[10] stressed that paramedical groups within the NHS should have access to library and information services in the same way that medical staff and nurse learners already had. Particular problems are posed by the comparatively small numbers of staff in one paramedical discipline in any hospital or health authority, and by the wide diversity of the literature. Library services should 'bring together literature from the biological, behavioural and social sciences' and 'take the initiative in disseminating the literature'.[10] In addition, it was thought that more attention should be given to the development of specialist current awareness bulletins and abstracting services. Chapter 3 of this book details progress in this field since 1985.

Brandon and Hill [18] were aware of the 'complexity and fractionation of the allied health literature' and that 'health sciences libraries frequently have "hit-or-miss" collections in the various allied health fields'. They considered that the development of information resources for this group should be considered to be as important as the development of similar resources for professions such as physicians, nurses or pharmacists, and that standard medical books and journals should be available to all allied health personnel.

Carmel[6] reviewed the UK scene briefly in 1986, and mentioned the need for: more library services to paramedical groups; access to a wider range of social information; and more visual and audio-visual information.

INFORMATION NEEDS OF PARAMEDICAL PERSONNEL

There has been little written on the information needs of paramedical staff. In 1977, Lloyd and Fraser[22] wrote on the information needs of physiotherapists in the

Atlantic provinces of Canada, and gave a brief guide to the books that should be included in a collection for physiotherapists in a small hospital. A second edition by Fraser and Lloyd in 1981 [484] expanded the guide to include some 600 items; these are now outdated, but the list is still a useful indication of the type of material that should be available to practising physiotherapists.

Research on the information needs of paramedical staff was carried out by Smith,[27] who studied the information needs of physiotherapists, the major paramedical group in Great Britain. She found that the most important sources of information were, in order, journals, colleagues at work, meetings, books and colleagues outside work. These were used primarily for keeping up to date and for clinical work. She recommended: more research on library services for physiotherapists, particularly on the extent of 'access to libraries of value' and the size of departmental collections; more research into the use of journals for current awareness rather than for reference; and a study of whether the literature base was 'as limited as has been suggested'.

Further work was carried out by Hewlett[17] into the needs for and use of information by paramedical staff and dentists in Haringey Health Authority. At the time (1985) there were no library services provided in the district for these groups of health care staff. The most heavily used sources were journals, colleagues at work, books and meetings, with many buying their own books and journals. About half the respondents made suggestions for library and information services, and for more provision of books or journals at the work-place.

The postal and telephone service supplied to paramedical and nursing staff in the Northern Regional Health Authority by Newcastle upon Tyne Polytechnic Library is well used, and usage is increasing. The service was reported soon after its inception by Walton et al.[30] and demand has shown no signs of levelling out. Information services provided include: literature searching; a current awareness service by monthly bulletin, either complete or partial; books on approval; and user education. The level of use appears to indicate that there is a real need, but that low use elsewhere might be related to poorer facilities and lack of access.

Much of the information provided to allied health staff is related to the information needs of the patient, and is often passed directly to them. Help for Health, a service of the Wessex Regional Library and Information Service, answered 6452 queries in 1985/86 on all aspects of patient information, of which 285 (4.4 per cent) were from the paramedical groups considered here.

INFORMATION AND THE ALLIED HEALTH PROFESSIONS

The literature of allied health between 1981 and 1988 was found by Brandon and Hill to be 'predominantly of practitioner quality' [18], although they were aware of considerable up-grading and expected that many allied health professionals would 'define both the theory and knowledge of their professions in their respective literatures' through scientific enquiry and research.

The professions have differing attitudes to information, in their awareness of what is available and how they can keep updated. In addition, there are different realizations of the need to publish and disseminate information, either as primary material or as secondary sources.

Chiropody

Chiropodists and podiatrists are aware of the need to keep updated, as Sumner[28] wrote in 1985. The *Journal of the American Podiatric Medical Association* [220] has a monthly column listing recent journal articles, by arrangement with the US National Library of Medicine. *The Chiropodist* [214], journal of the (British) Society of Chiropodists, has considered such a service but does not supply it.[7]

Occupational Therapy

The literature of occupational therapy has been cumulated in a number of bibliographies, covering the years from 1895, which have allowed scope for citation analysis by Johnson and Leising.[18] They found that the literature depended to a large extent on that of other disciplines. Reed[26] has analysed the US serial sources of occupational therapy articles, with similar results. She has also written on the need for researchers' access to the literature,[25] and Kelly has written for a British audience on keeping up to date with journals.[19] Hall[16] has discussed ten databases that cover rehabilitation to some extent.

Physiotherapy

Physiotherapists, perhaps the largest group, are aware of the need to keep updated and to have regular access to published material, as Arnell shows.[1] In addition, their literature contains material on how to use libraries, by Bunch[5]; how to find relevant references, by Bohannon[2]; how to store them, by Lehmkuhl[21] and Mater[23]; and how to evaluate research literature, by Domholdt and Malone.[11] Library orientation programmes have been researched by Williams *et al.*[31] and the clinical use made of information on new practices by Fuhrer and Grabois.[13]

Dietetics, Radiography and Speech Therapy

The literature of the three other paramedical disciplines of dietetics, radiography and speech therapy covered here does not appear to have excited the same interest. The reasons are imponderable, but may be in part because of their relationship to other disciplines: dietetics and nutrition are closely related to physiology, a pre-clinical medical science; speech therapy is related to education; radiography is perhaps considered as within the medical literature, linked with radiology and radiotherapy.

References

1. Arnell, P. (1985). Awareness of and access to physiotherapy-related publications: a professional necessity. *Physiotherapy*, **71** (6), 271.
2. Bohannon, R. (1988). How to find relevant references for a publication. *Physiotherapy Practice*, **4** (1), 41–4.
3. Brember, G. and Leggate, P. (1982). Matching user needs in health care. *Aslib Proceedings*, **34** (2), 90–102.
4. *British Medical Journal* (1982). Briefing: professions supplementary to medicine. *British Medical Journal*, **284**, 680–1.
5. Bunch, A. J. (1980). Using libraries. *Physiotherapy*, **66**, 337–9.
6. Carmel, M. J. (1986). Users of biomedical libraries. *Health Libraries Review*, **3** (1), 28–34.
7. *Chiropodist* (Editorial) (1985). Articles in the medical press. *Chiropodist*, **40** (7), 235.
8. Clark, K. (1984). The library needs of the paramedical professions: a workshop report of a seminar held on 18th October, 1983. *Library Association, Nursing Interest Sub-Group Newsletter*, **4** (1), 5–6.
9. Council for Professions Supplementary to Medicine (1988). *Annual report of the Council for Professions Supplementary to Medicine, 1987–88*. London: CPSM.
10. Department of Health and Social Security and NHS Regional Librarians' Group, Joint Working Party on Library Services (1985). *Providing a district library service*. Proposals arising from a series of workshops held in 1983 about the contribution library services can make to the provision and use of information in the NHS. London: King's Fund Centre.
11. Domholdt, E. A. and Malone, T. R. (1985). Evaluating research literature: the education clinician. *Physical Therapy*, **65**, 487–91.
12. Donald, B. (1978). Professions auxiliary, supplementary or complementary to medicine. *Health Trends*, **10**, 5–9.
13. Fuhrer, M. J. and Grabois, M. (1988). Information sources that influence physiatrists' adoption of new clinical practices. *Archives of Physical Medicine and Rehabilitation*, **69** (3), 167–9.
14. Great Britain, Statutes (1954). *National Health Service (medical auxiliaries) regulations 1954*. SI 1954, no. 55. London: HMSO.
15. Great Britain, Statutes (1960). Professions Supplementary to Medicine Act 1960. London: HMSO.
16. Hall, M. (1987). Unlocking information technology. *American Journal of Occupational Therapy*, **41** (11), 722–5.
17. Hewlett, J. F. (1986). Information needs of paramedical staff and dental workers in Haringey Health Authority. MSc (Information Science) thesis, The City University, London.
18. Johnson, K. S. and Leising, D. J. (1986). The literature of occupational therapy: a citation analysis study. *American Journal of Occupational Therapy*, **40**, 390–6.

19. Kelly, G. (1987). Keeping up with the journals. *British Journal of Occupational Therapy*, **50** (9), 289–99.
20. Larkin, G. (1983). *Occupational monopoly and modern medicine*. London: Tavistock Publications. 212 pp.
21. Lehmkuhl, D. (1978). Techniques for locating, filing and retrieving scientific information. *Physical Therapy*, **58**, 579–84.
22. Lloyd, H. A. and Fraser, M. D. E. (1977). *Information needs of physiotherapists in the Atlantic Provinces, with suggested physiotherapy working collections for small hospitals*. Halifax, Nova Scotia: Dalhousie University School of Library Science. 39 pp.
23. Mater, D. A. (1986). Managing your personal information files. *Physical and Occupational Therapy in Pediatrics*, **6**, 95–101.
24. Ministry of Health and Department of Health for Scotland (1951). *Reports of the Committees on Medical Auxiliaries*: V. Z. Cope, chairman. (Cmnd 8188.) London: HMSO. 25 pp.
25. Reed, K. (1987). Access to literature is basic to research. *American Journal of Occupational Therapy*, **41** (11), 761–3.
26. Reed, K. L. (1988). Occupational therapy articles in serial publications: an analysis of sources. *Bulletin of the Medical Library Association*, **76** (2), 125–30.
27. Smith, D. L. (1978). The information needs of physiotherapists. MA (Information Studies) thesis, Sheffield University.
28. Sumner, R. (1985). Keeping up to date (letter). *Chiropodist*, **40** (10), 346.
29. Tabor, R. B., ed. (1973). *Information and library services in the NHS: Wessex research project*. Southampton: Wessex Regional Library and Information Service.
30. Walton, J. G., Bailey, P., Bond, S. and Cook, A. M. (1982). The provision of a library and information service to Northern Regional Health Authority trained nursing and paramedical staff by Newcastle-upon-Tyne Polytechnic. *Aslib Proceedings*, **34** (8), 364–71.
31. Williams, R., Baker, L. and Roberts, J. G. (1987). Information searching in health care: a pilot study. *Physiotherapy Canada*, **39** (2), 102–9.

2 Finding Out about the Literature

John Hewlett

USING LIBRARIES AND LITERATURE

Guides to Using the Literature

Guides to using the literature outline the major sources of information, either printed or otherwise, and may contain bibliographies of relevant books, periodicals and other materials. They may also contain guidance on how to search the literature to obtain further information, and how to use libraries.

The most useful brief guide to the literature is probably Barbara Smith's *Sources of information on remedial health* [1], written for 'physiotherapy and occupational therapy students and for those about to embark on research in these fields'. This has very helpful information about using libraries, and discusses information sources and relevant databases. It also contains a bibliography, divided into sections covering remedial health disciplines and therapeutic skills respectively. She reminds her readers that 'remedial health information is not neatly packaged and organised with exactly your problem in mind', a statement that will be taken to heart by most allied health staff.

An earlier useful work is *Health studies: a guide to the sources of information* [2]. This was written as part of a package which included video and tape–slide programmes, for students on Newcastle Polytechnic's Health Studies course; it outlines how to find information in health studies and the different types of literature. The Open University course P251, The handicapped person in the community, ceased in 1988; Dale's helpful *Guide to using the literature* [3] has been obtainable as a module of Course E241, Special needs in education, but in 1990 that course also ends.

(There are proposals to replace both courses but details are unknown at present.)

Other books aiming to show the health care worker how to trace literature are written for the medical user. The general information is equally relevant for the allied health professional, with examples taken from the medical literature. Strickland-Hodge and Allan produced *Medical information: a profile* [6] as a practical guide to medical sources, with good detail on online services. *How to search the medical sources*, by Livesey and Strickland-Hodge [6a], is limited and less useful on paramedical subjects, although it is still helpful for medical and pharmaceutical sources. Welch and King's *Searching the medical literature: a guide to published and online sources* [7] gives more detail on searching for information.

The *British Medical Journal* has issued two compilations of articles entitled *How to do it*. The second of these [9] includes chapters by J. Stephen on 'How to search the literature' (pp. 77–82) and 'How to carry out an online search' (pp. 83–6), which are basic reading for anyone doing studies or research in any health care field. A similar volume for nurses in *Guide to nursing literature*, by Binger and Jensen [10]. This has helpful advice on literature searching and keeping updated, with a list of reference sources. Jenkins's *Medical libraries* [4] is a brief practical guide to how a medical library serves its users, with a particularly good section on journals.

Guides to Using Libraries

Medical libraries: a user guide, by Stan Jenkins [4], was written for the centenary of the British Medical Association in 1987. It is a brief, readable guide, giving a good outline of how a medical library serves its users. A similar older book by Morton and Wright, *How to use a medical library* [5], has a new edition.

The first *How to do it* [8] compilation from the *British Medical Journal* included a chapter on 'How to use a library' by Timbury (pp. 183–7). Strickland-Hodge and Allan's *Medical information* [6] includes a brief section on libraries. Binger and Jensen's *Guide to nursing literature* [10] has helpful advice on using (American) libraries. Most librarians produce some form of guide to their services, and are always willing to assist by answering questions and advising on their own library's use.

Finding a Library

Library funding in the UK may be for specific user groups, such as doctors or nurse learners, rather than for all health care staff. This may result in a local NHS library not offering services to all user groups, so that allied health staff are without a full library service. Library staff are aware of this but may not have the time to offer services to clients outside their terms of reference. More information on NHS libraries locally is obtainable from the Regional Librarian, or the regional representative on the Regional Librarians' Group: addresses are given in Part III of this book. Public libraries will also be able to help, although they will have little specialist material, and obtaining items from elsewhere might take a little time; however, they will have better collections of general reference materials than most local NHS libraries.

The Library Association's *Directory of medical and health care libraries in the UK and Republic of Ireland* [11] lists 604 libraries by location. It does not list libraries that *contain* health care materials, so it gives few polytechnic or general university libraries, although these may contain collections on, for example, dietetics or speech therapy. Heap's *Sources of information for therapists* [12] is a brief guide to NHS postgraduate centre libraries that might be open to therapists. The *Aslib directory of information sources in the UK*; vol. 2, *Social sciences, medicine and the humanities* [13] lists information sources of all kinds; these do not all have libraries or supply information to all.

In the USA, the Medical Library Association's *Directory of health sciences libraries* [14] is irregularly produced, and lists US libraries that deal with health sciences subjects. Backus's *Medical and health information directory* [152] lists US libraries in volume 2. Jaeggin [15] has written briefly on the network of libraries in Canada offering resources on disability, which will be of use to health care personnel in that country.

GENERAL INFORMATION SOURCES

Walford's *Guide to reference materials* [16] and Sheehy's *Guide to reference books* [17] are the British and American guides to the major reference materials in all subjects. Their coverage overlaps to a great extent, and both can usually be found in large public reference libraries. Walford [16] is issued in three volumes: volume 1 covers science, technology and medicine, but the fourth edition of 1980 is the latest for this volume. Sheehy [17] is a single volume, last issued in 1986. For general subjects these are both invaluable, but where more detailed works are required, specialist information sources should be consulted.

HEALTH CARE INFORMATION SOURCES

Brandon and Hill's 'Selected list of books and journals in allied health sciences' was published in the *Bulletin of the Medical Library Association* in October 1988 [18]; previous lists had appeared in 1986 [19] and 1984 [20]. This listed 435 books and 76 journals on all aspects of allied health sciences, under broad subjects, and included some 207 books and 42 periodicals on dietetics, radiography and related sciences, physiotherapy, occupational therapy and rehabilitation. There is a very good section on terminology, largely American. Brandon and Hill is kept up to date by *A Major Report* [27], a quarterly newsletter from Majors Scientific Books [1302].

The major British guide to the literature of medicine is Morton and Godbolt's

Information sources in the medical sciences [28]. This is an invaluable reference source for general medical materials, arranged by type of material. Smith [1], Cook *et al.* [2] and Strickland-Hodge and Allan [6] all include sections of references to printed sources of information, although that in the latter is largely medical.

Chen's work on *Health sciences information sources* [21] is intended for librarians and has a strong medical emphasis. It is arranged by type of material with detailed author and title indexes, but without a subject index. Roper and Boorkman's *Introduction to reference sources in the health sciences* [30] is arranged by broad subject headings and was written for library school students, but is sometimes useful for library users. Kurian's *Global guide to medical information* [26] is arranged by type of information and is good on databases and publishers, but not as helpful for paramedical periodicals or associations.

Government publications are often difficult to trace and to locate, although the health care field is easier than some others. British government sources are briefly covered in the HMSO *Medicine and health catalogue* [24], Less descriptive are the British HMSO sectional lists for the Department of Health and Social Security [23], which in 1988 divided into separate Departments, of Health and of Social Security, and the Office of Population Censuses and Surveys [25]. Other British guides are covered in [105]–[110]. A useful bibliography of US federal publications on health and medicine has been compiled by Chitty and Schatz, who list some 1300 items [29]. A briefer guide to US government sources for nursing and health information can be found in *Reference services review*, published in 1984 [29a].

Self reviews over 1000 works on physical handicap in her *Physical disability: an annotated literature guide* [31]. This comprehensive survey of material selected on the basis of availability, quality, uniqueness, audience and significance in the field also includes notes on some 60 journals relevant to disability. More recent references on specific aspects of disability can be found in the Disabled Living Foundation's *Information service handbook* [156], issued in 24 sections. Each section contains a list of recent publications (as well as lists of equipment and addresses); for example, section 6 on 'leisure activities' lists some 110 publications.

The *Health information handbook* by Gann [22] is based on the innovative work of Help for Health in the Wessex Regional Health Authority, which was established as a resource centre for health consumers when health began to be seen more as a responsibility of the 'patient'. Gann looks at information sources for self-care, and there are useful references and lists of other resource centres.

PERIODICALS

Periodicals are the major primary source of information on research-based disciplines. As the paramedical professions have evolved, there is now a greater emphasis on research and dissemination of the results of this research, with a consequent growth in the number of both major and minor periodicals in the field.

Periodicals (or serials or journals) appear in a variety of guises: 'pure' research journals, containing only research results; publications of a society or association, which contain research papers and include meeting reports and news; newsletters and newspapers that aim to keep readers up to date with what is happening in the profession; and commercially sponsored journals, which rely heavily on advertising and may be free. All these types of periodical contain information, but due consideration should be given to the quality and status of the periodical where the information appears. Medical periodicals such as *British Medical Journal*, *Lancet* and *New England Journal of Medicine* will often have articles relevant to allied health, as will journals for health care management and administration, such as *Health Service Journal*.

There are few paramedical journals that cover all the disciplines included here. *Journal of Allied Health* [46] is published quarterly by the American Society of Allied Health Professions (ASAHP), and is now in its sixteenth year: it contains original articles, book reviews and occasional abstracts of relevant articles published elsewhere. ASAHP includes a wide range of allied health disciplines, and also issues a monthly newsletter, *Trends* [54]. *Therapy Weekly* [53] is a 'newspaper for the remedial professions' giving news, new-product information, brief meeting reports and job advertisements. It has a largely free circulation to NHS staff in the UK.

There are many periodical titles on general rehabilitation that cover material of interest to allied health professions, such as *Clinical Rehabilitation* [41], *International Journal of Rehabilitation Research* [45], and *American Archives of Rehabilitation Therapy* [33]. Some of these are written by medical authors rather than paramedical authors, such as *International Disability Studies* [44] and *Scandinavian Journal of Rehabilitation Medicine* [52]. There are also titles on specific therapies, such as *British Journal of Music Therapy* [40] and *American Journal of Dance Therapy* [36].

Periodicals Directories

Periodicals directories can be used to find out what periodicals exist in your chosen subject; who are the publishers; which services index or abstract them; their frequency and cost; and where you can see the original or obtain a photocopy of an article.

The major directory of serials is *Ulrich's International periodicals directory* [57], published in alternate years. It is a list of some 111 000 current periodical titles, arranged in broad subject groups; some 400 allied health titles are listed under a variety of headings. There are descriptions for some 10 000 titles, and all have an indication of their contents, their current price, publisher and address, and where they are indexed or abstracted. They are indexed by title and subject, and there are also lists of new and ceased titles, and an index by International Standard Serial Number (ISSN). *Ulrich* is also available on microfiche for a subscription, revised quarterly, and annually on a CD-ROM.

Medical and Health Care Books and Serials in Print [113] contains a useful list of medical and health care periodicals. They are arranged by broad subject, but not always by the most obvious subject; for example, physiotherapy titles are included under 'medical scineces' and chiropody titles under 'surgery'. But they are traceable through the subject index, and full details are given, as in *Ulrich*. The British Library (BL) publishes a quarterly *Keyword Index to Serial Titles* or *KIST* [55], which lists BL (and other libraries') holdings by all significant words in the titles and gives their locations. It covers all subjects. The annual *List of Journals Indexed in Index Medicus* [56] is issued separately from *Index Medicus* and is available from the USGPO. All titles are listed four times, by abbreviated title, full title, subject and country of origin.

Another type of periodicals directory is the union list of serials, which gives information on titles and holdings of participating libraries. These are usually tools for librarians, but may be used by readers on occasion, for example, when visiting another library to consult periodicals. The local librarian will have access to such lists, whether local, regional or national.

Indexes and Abstracts

Indexes and abstracts are used to find what periodical articles have been published, either on specific subjects or by specific authors. Indexes list the source of the article only, and abstracts include a brief abstract or precis of the article. They both contain enough information to identify the article and its periodical source; this usually includes author(s), title of article, title of periodical, date of issue, volume, part and page numbers; it may also include authors address(es), standard periodical abbreviation, periodical coden or ISSN. Indexes and abstracts may cover general subjects or be very specific.

The major indexing and abstracting services in the medical and health care field are covered in more detail in Chapter 3. They are *Index Medicus* [58] and *Excerpta Medica* [65], which deal with medicine in its widest sense, the *Cumulative Index to Nursing and Allied Health Literature (CINAHL)* [69] and *Health Service Abstracts* [71]. Sutherland lists some 40 sources in his chapter on abstracts, indexes and bibliographies in Morton and Godbolt [28].

Indexes to the rehabilitation literature include the *International Bibliographical Documentation on Rehabilitation*, now contained in *Clinical Rehabilitation* [41], which is published quarterly in Heidelberg. It lists rehabilitation literature by subject, including rehabilitation of the physically handicapped, of the speech and hearing impaired, and so on. A very wide range of journals is covered, but the index is rather limited, which makes retrospective searching difficult. An annual review of rehabilitation literature is produced in Chicago, *Year Book of Rehabilitation* [94]. This reviews some 110 journals, mainly in occupational therapy, physical therapy and medicine; arrangement is by subject. *Rehabilitation Literature* [93], which ceased publication in 1986, was a useful source of information on the rehabilitation of handicapped children and adults.

Health care management and administration are covered by four services. *Health Service Abstracts* [71] is discussed in Chapter 3. The other British source is

HELMIS: Health Management Information Service [87], produced at the Nuffield Institute for Health Service Studies. This is available at various levels, from a monthly current awareness bulletin only up to online access to the database. It was described soon after its inception by Perry.[8] *Hospital Literature Index* [88] is produced quarterly by the American Hospital Association (AHA), and is cumulated in the fourth quarter; this cumulation is also available on microfiche. It covers management literature, arranged by *MeSH* headings [60] with an author index. Each annual cumulation also includes a list of recent acquisitions by the Library of the AHA, some 900 titles in 1987. The annual *Abstracts of Health Care Management Studies* [85] is not as comprehensive as *Hospital Literature Index* but has very informative abstracts. These two sources should be used together to find information, particularly on American aspects.

Social sciences indexes and abstracts are used to obtain information on the social and community aspects of health care. The widest coverage of British materials is found in *ASSIA, Applied Social Sciences Indexes and Abstracts* [86], which is produced six times a year by the Library Association; it indexes some 550 international titles, and arranges material by subject. The author index gives the reference with subject heading so that the abstract can be found, and is cumulated annually. Narrower in scope is *Social Service Abstracts* [73], produced with *Health Service Abstracts* [71] and also forming part of the online *DHSS-Data* [99] (see Chapter 3). It includes some 240 citations a month, arranged by subject, and is particularly useful for occupational therapists, physiotherapists and speech therapists. Subject and author indexes are detailed and cumulated monthly.

Nursing indexes are useful sources of information on the edge of the allied health field, containing general health care references as well as nursing material. *International Nursing Index* [89] is a quarterly listing of articles from over 270 nursing journals, with additional material. It is arranged by *MeSH* [60] subjects with author indexes and can be searched online using *Medline* [101]. The Royal College of Nursing's *Nursing Bibliography* [90] is produced monthly and cumulated annually, and indexes some 120 journals with additional material. A particularly useful aspect is the cumulations, available in four volumes covering 1959 to 1980 [91]. *Nursing Research Abstracts* [72] is produced quarterly by the Department of Health Library with an annual cumulated index, and lists British research in nursing, either published or in progress.

ONLINE DATABASES AND DATABANKS

Online databases are the computerized equivalent of a printed or abstract journal, containing indexed bibliographic references. They can be searched online using a computer (or computer terminal) and a telecommunications link. Database producers make them available through database vendors, who can offer different databases and facilities. A useful guide to the variety of commands has been produced by Arthur [95]. Databases likely to be relevant to health care are listed by Farbey [96] and include *CINAHL* [97], *DHSS-Data* [99], *EMBase* [100], *Medline* [101] and others. More information on all of these is given in Chapter 3.

Databanks contain factual information rather than bibliographic references. They are less used in health care at present, other than in administration and medical records management [205]. For example, *BARDSOFT* [421] contains copies of software programs available from a variety of sources for people with special rehabilitation needs of all kinds. More databanks of this kind are being developed, as more people become aware of the potential uses of computers.

BIBLIOGRAPHIES

Bibliographies can be used for purposes similar to those of periodical indexes and abstracts, to find what has been published on a specific subject or by a particular author. They may be general or subject-specific; international, national or language-specific; and published singly or updated regularly. The information included may not be very detailed, or it may include all information about the book as well as annotations on the contents.

The major general bibliographies are *Whitaker's Books in Print* and *Books in Print*. *Whitaker's Books in Print* [102] now lists more than 90 per cent of books published and on sale in the UK, listed in a single sequence of authors/editors/titles; additional title keywords are also used to help with the location of items. Publishers are listed with their address. *Whitaker's* is available either as four annual bound volumes or as microfiche, replaced monthly. *Books in Print* [103] is issued annually by Bowker, and lists all the books printed and available in the USA. The 1988/89 volumes include references to some 800 000 books, listed by author and title in the first three volumes; Volumes 4–7 contain the subject guide to non-fiction books (some 675 000 titles) listed by subject. There is also a mid-year update in two volumes, with over 45 000 titles in 1988; and six bi-monthly issues for forthcoming books, containing about 85 000 titles each year. *Books in Print* is also obtainable on microfiche, completely updated every quarter.

Another useful bibliography is *Books at Boston Spa* or *BABS* [104], issued in alternate months on microfiche by the British Library. This lists some 250 000 books published since 1979, 90 per cent in English, and is invaluable for checking information; the material is arranged by author/editor and title, but there is no subject listing.

Access to information on government publications other than in health care can be obtained by using the HMSO catalogues and lists [105]–[107] and Chadwyck-Healey's *British Official Publications Not Published by HMSO* [108]; the latter complements the former by listing more than 50 per cent of British government publications. They are cumulated together as *United Kingdom Official Publications* (*UKOP*) [109], containing information on CD-ROM from 1980 to date; there is a useful brief guide to government publications in general [109a]. Richard's

Directory of British official publications [110] is now in its second edition and is a helpful (though brief) guide to general sources.

Medical Bibliographies

Medical and Health Care Books and Serials in Print [113] is an annual listing, by author and title, of English language books in print in the USA (and therefore available in the UK); a second volume contains the subject index and a list of periodicals. Full details are given, including publisher, price (in dollars), pages and ISBN. There is a complete address list of publishers.

The National Library of Medicine issues its catalogue in two forms, as hard copy and as microfiche. The *NLM Current Catalog* [118] is a hard copy quarterly, with annual cumulations; it is arranged by subject using *MeSH* [60] and by author, with an additional section of reference works listed by *MeSH* subject. The *NLM Catalog* [116] is issued as microfiche; the 1984 edition contained nearly 600 000 items on 796 fiche, and each subsequent quarterly supplement [117] supersedes previous supplements. They are available as an annual subscription, or the December issue can be obtained singly.

A major bibliography covering the medical and health sciences was cumulated from the computer and hard copy information in *Medical and Health Care Books and Serials in Print* and issued in four volumes in 1982 as *Health science books, 1876–1982* [111]. This includes three volumes of subject listing and a fourth of very good author and title indexes. Unfortunately the subject listing is variable, with books being listed, for example, under 'chiropody' or 'foot' or 'podiatry'.

Leslie Morton's *A medical bibliography* [114] is a meticulously prepared list of texts illustrating the history of medicine, listing historical and classic materials by subject. It includes references to first descriptions of diseases and their treatment, and has detailed indexes.

The National Library of Medicine also issues two bibliographies of audio-visual materials. *Health Sciences Audiovisuals* [112] is a quarterly, on microfiche, with each issue updating previous issues, and covering 1975 to date. It is arranged by *MeSH* subjects and author/title, with lists of sources and serials indexes. *NLM Audiovisuals Catalog* [115] contains only the new information, and the quarterly hard copy issues are cumulated annually.

CONFERENCES AND PROCEEDINGS

Tracing conference proceedings and papers can be a difficult task, but three major tools make it much easier. The British Library's *Index of Conference Proceedings* [119] is issued monthly with an annual cumulation, and contains details of about 1500 conferences each month. It is arranged by subject, using keywords from the title of the conference. Full details of the conference are given, including the BL location, which is useful for borrowing. Cumulations published include 1964–81 on microfiche, and the whole index is available online as *Conference Proceedings Index* [98].

The Institute for Scientific Information publishes two indexes that list the articles in the proceedings. The *Index to Scientific and Technical Proceedings* [120] is issued monthly, and the *Index to Social Sciences and Humanities Proceedings* [121] appears quarterly. These are both cumulated annually and indexed by conference topic, title keywords, author/editor, sponsor, location of conference and corporate address (giving addresses of authors). A brief review of the US sources by Brahmi[1] looks at some of the major published and online sources of conference proceedings information.

DICTIONARIES

Dictionaries can be selected by considering their coverage, their authority (which includes their history, editors and the reference sources used), their arrangement and their modernity. They are helpfully outlined by Hague in Morton and Godbolt [28], and further information can be found there.

The largest current medical dictionary is the *Wiley International dictionary of medicine and biology* [142], in three volumes. It has a very wide range of subjects, indexing single words rather than compound terms, and grouping compound terms under their parts, such as 'position' and 'therapy'. Another broad dictionary is the *Encyclopedia and dictionary of medicine, nursing and allied health* [134], edited by Miller and Keane. This usefully includes many paramedical terms not easily found in other purely medical dictionaries. Kamenetz compiled his *Dictionary of rehabilitation medicine* [131] because 'only part of its terminology can be found in any one medical dictionary'. It groups terms such as 'exercise' and 'position', and includes abbreviations such as ASHA and CSP, although these are often given no further clarification (such as British or American origin). The same author produced a translating dictionary, rare in this field, the *English–French dictionary of physical medicine and rehabilitation* [132], published in 1972 with its French–English equivalent [133].

In a closely related field is Tver and Hunt's recent *Encyclopedic dictionary of sports medicine* [141], particularly useful for physiotherapists. The Council of Europe has produced *Rehabilitation of disabled persons: glossary and list of the principal terms* [126], which is a short guide to terminology in this field. Schmidt's *Paramedical dictionary* [136] is rather dated now, but can still be helpful.

The major British medical dictionary is *Butterworth's Medical dictionary* [127], its second edition in 1978 establishing it as the authoritative work. It contains simple definitions and some longer entries; there are compound terms grouped together, such as 'diet' and 'joint'; eponymous terms are included under the originator's names, with brief biographical details and references from the compound term. It also contains some 80 pages of anatomical nomenclature. *Baillière's Encyclopaedic dictionary of nursing and health care* [121a] and *Churchill's Illustrated medical dictionary*

[122a] are new British publications in this field. Smaller British works are the *Heinemann Medical dictionary* [130] and the Oxford *Concise medical dictionary* [124], which is 'intended primarily for workers in the paramedical fields'.

There are five major American medical dictionaries, of comparable size. The choice between them will depend on personal preference, although they are rarely available together in one library. *Dorland's Illustrated medical dictionary* [128], sometimes considered as the standard American medical text, reached its 27th edition in 1988. *Mosby's Medical and nursing dictionary* [135] is the newest of the five, its second edition having been published in 1986. *Taber's Cyclopedic medical dictionary* [140] is aimed primarily at nurses and allied health staff, averaging an edition every three years from 1940 to 1989. The 24th edition of *Stedman's Medical dictionary* [137] was published in 1982, and includes a useful section on medical etymology. *Blakiston's Gould medical dictionary* [122] is now the oldest, its fourth edition being dated 1979, but it has the longest history, dating originally from 1890. Callard and Fruehauf[2] compared older editions of these dictionaries in 1978, giving more details about their style and information. There are also two useful smaller American medical dictionaries: *Stedman's Pocket medical dictionary*, 1987, [138] and *Dorland's Pocket medical dictionary*, 1982 [129].

Clegg's *Dictionary of social services policy and practice* [123] is another specific dictionary, with definitions of all aspects of social services, and comments on policies and practices. *Sweet and Maxwell's Encyclopaedia of health services and medical law* [139] is an invaluable loose-leaf compendium, updated regularly, which contains British statutes and statutory instruments and summarizes EEC law. There is a good introduction to the subject and a very detailed subject index. This is the only source that brings together all the relevant material. The Council of Europe has produced *Legislation on the rehabilitation of disabled people in thirteen member states* [125], which brings together all the relevant legislation.

Eponyms, Syndromes and Nomenclature

The use of personal names has been widespread in medicine from the earliest times, but often needs definition and clarification. People's names provide convenient short-hand for therapies (Fisk's splint), for parts of the anatomy (Achilles tendon) or for pathological states (Osgood–Schlatter syndrome). There are useful guides to the pathological states and syndromes, but the usual dictionaries must be used for many anatomical and therapy terms.

A second edition of Jablonski's *Dictionary of syndromes and eponymic diseases* [143] was published in 1990, 20 years after the first edition; it is well illustrated and arranged by personal name. Magalini and Scrascia's *Dictionary of medical syndromes* [145] is perhaps more comprehensive, and is arranged in the same way, but with more information on symptoms, diagnosis, therapy and prognosis. A briefer outline with some 900 entries is *Medical eponyms: who was Coude?* [144], with short biographical outlines. Firkin and Whitworth have recently written on eponyms used in Australian internal medicine in their *Dictionary of medical eponyms* [146].

The terminology of medicine and related subjects is complex, but clarified by a number of authors. *Medical terminology* by Davies [147] is largely clinical and medical, but with a very good introduction and a useful index; Roberts's *Medical terms: their origin and construction* [149] shows clearly how terms are derived from their sources; and Rickards's *Understanding medical terms: a self-instructional course* [148] is one of a number of essentially similar self-programmed texts, written for new students of health care.

Abbreviations in medicine by Steen [150] is of limited use for allied health subjects. It is very good on medical terms, but does not include ASAHP, ASHA or COT, and BDA is given as the British Dental Association only. Strauss's *Familiar medical quotations* [151] is useful for tracing quotations for speeches or when writing, including such statements as 'the right way of looking at things will see through anything' (on X-rays).

DIRECTORIES

Directories included in this section can be used to find information on hospitals and health care services, societies and people in the allied health professions.

The major British directory in the field is the *Hospitals and health service yearbook* [161], issued annually by the Institute of Health Services Management. This is arranged by Regional Health Authority, subdivided to give information on District Health Authorities and hospitals. It also contains lists of statutory instruments and health circulars, summaries of major reports since 1954, and a very useful bibliography on the NHS. The annual *Directory of hospitals* [154] is a smaller alphabetical list, divided into state and independent hospitals. It is indexed by health authority or board, by hospital type and by town. It is useful to have one listing of all UK hospitals together. There is also a British *Directory of independent hospitals and health services* [155], which contains separate lists of different private health services, each arranged geographically or by health authority or board in each section.

Backus's *Medical and health information directory* [152] contains largely American information in three volumes. Volume 1 contains information on associations (international, national and state) and medical and allied health schools (including dietetics, occupational therapy, physiotherapy, podiatry, rehabilitation and respiratory therapy). Volume 2 lists publications and other information sources, including sections on periodicals, abstracts and indexes, audiovisual media, computerized information services (all international) and libraries (US only). Volume 3 lists American health services. All three volumes are very well indexed.

Kruzas's *Encyclopedia of medical organizations and agencies* [163] contains some 10 000 entries in 78 subject chapters, each divided into eight sections including national and international associations, state government agencies and research centres and institutes. It is more 'medical' than the newer *Encyclopedia of health information sources* [166] edited by Wasserman, and also published by Gale. This includes some 13 000 information sources, again largely American, in 450 subject divisions. The lack of an index makes this difficult to use, particularly with some subject areas, such as speech and hearing disorders.

There is one biographical directory in the field, *Who's who in rehabilitation* [167], which lists people in three sections: medical graduates, basic scientists and researchers, and associated professionals. There are useful indexes by clinical emphasis, by research emphasis and by occupation.

The *Social services yearbook* [165] contains a wide range of information on all aspects of social services, such as: legal aspects; government departments; health authorities; advice and counselling centres; education and training. There is a listing of social service media (which includes some 250 journal titles in 1989/90) and a bibliography.

The Disabled Living Foundation produces its *Information service handbook* [156] on a rolling programme, updating each of its 24 sections annually. It can be obtained as a bi-monthly bulletin of four updated sections, and single sections are purchasable for a nominal cost. The handbook is particularly relevant for occupational therapists, physiotherapists and speech therapists, although other health care professionals will find it useful. Each section lists recent relevant publications, the equipment, and addresses of publishers and suppliers; for example, Section 13 on 'pressure relief', has 35 references and 130 addresses, in addition to descriptions of equipment.

The series *Equipment for the disabled* [157] lists, evaluates and illustrates the same range of equipment, and each of its 12 sections is regularly updated; for example, the 'communications' section is now in its sixth edition, published in 1987. The *Directory for disabled people* by Darnborough and Kinrade [153] is now in its fifth edition, and includes a wide range of UK information. It covers aid centres, organizations and statutory services, and contains a list of publications on a range of needs and activities for people with disabilities, with a very good index. Hale's *New source book for the disabled* [158], in contrast, is well illustrated and more for the general reader. It is rather dated now, but still useful. A useful brief list of UK disabled living centres that can provide information is given by Chamberlain,[3] and another list of resource centres on infant health and development is given by Cochrane and Mater.[4] Similar lists of resource centres on specific subjects appear regularly in the periodical press.

Robertson's *Disability rights handbook* [164] covers the rights, benefits and services for the 3.5 million disabled in the UK and their families. *Aids and adaptations* by Keeble [162] looks at the administrative processes by which social services departments help clients to receive aid and adaptations to their homes.

The most comprehensive directory to societies is by Zeitak and Berman, *Directory of international and national medical and related societies* [168]. They are listed by country, in an international section, and indexed by society title and by broad subject; only brief details are given. *The Directory of British associations and associations in Ireland* [160] gives very full information about some 6000 associations and societies in the British Isles, listed in alphabetical order with a very detailed subject index.

GUIDES TO RESEARCH

Allied health disciplines are becoming more research oriented, and more postgraduate theses and dissertations are being produced. *Journal of Allied Health* [46] has produced an index of graduate theses and projects annually since 1979. This contained 415 items in 1987, under 23 headings that included a wide range of allied health disciplines (though not chiropody). At present it includes only American theses and dissertations, although a single international list would be useful. A wider coverage is obtained from the *Aslib Index to Theses* [169], issued annually until 1975 and then twice a year. Titles are arranged by 74 major and over 300 minor subjects, and indexed by author and by selected keywords.

Dissertation Abstracts International [171] is published in three parts: A, *Humanities and Social Sciences* appears monthly; B, *Sciences and Engineering* also appears monthly; C, *European Dissertations* appears quarterly. Each section lists dissertations under broad subject groups, with an abstract written by the author, and indexing is by title keywords and authors. Sections A and B are available on microfiche, and also available annually on microfiche in sections such as 'health and environmental sciences' and 'social sciences'.

Research in progress is covered by *Current Research in Britain* [170], produced by the British Library. The volumes on *Social Sciences* and *Biological Sciences* are the most relevant to allied health care. They are arranged by institution, and indexed by researcher's name, by subject studied (in broad groups and narrower divisions) and by detailed subject keyword. Regular updating means that research listed here is in progress rather than completed. It is also available online.

A similar volume, though older, is the *Medical research directory* [173], which arranges research projects by broad subject groups, and indexes them by name and by specific topic. *Medical research centres* [172] is an international guide to institutions doing research on a subject area rather than to specific research projects, and therefore indexes them under general terms, such as 'physiotherapy', rather than 'stroke' or 'dynamometry'.

GUIDES TO STATISTICS

Statistical information is more easily traced and two useful guides to it are by Anne Cowie and Welch and King. Cowie [175] describes UK and some international sources, and gives lists arranged by subject, as well as useful addresses. Welch and King [7] cover international sources and give items for futher reading. The Central Statistical Office's *Guide to official statistics* [174] is published in alternate years and gives a readable introduction to a wide range of UK statistics, particularly on 'population and vital statistics' and 'social statistics' in Chapters 3 and 4.

Major British sources of statistical information are *Health and Personal Social Services Statistics for England* [176] and *Scottish Health Statistics* [180]. Both cover similar health administration fields, but the latter has more detailed tables; for example, of chiropody patients and treatments and of mass radiography figures. Also useful is the annual *Social Trends* [181], which covers population, households and families, and such social aspects as housing. The Office of Population Censuses and Surveys (OPCS) publishes more detailed statistics as *OPCS Monitors* [177] for the quick release of information, and the cumulated *OPCS Reference Series* [178], which may be annual or less regular. A new series is the *OPCS Surveys of Disablity in Great Britain* [179]; one of the recent issues looks at the financial circumstances of disabled adults.

Full information on British government statistical publications can be obtained from the HMSO catalogues and lists [105]–[107], Chadwyck-Healey's *British Official Publications Not Published by HMSO* [108] and their joint publication *UKOP* [109].

HOW TO DO IT: RESEARCH AND STATISTICS

Starting work in research involves a wide variety of different systems and methods, such as raising funds, applying for research grants and planning research projects, as well as writing up the results of the research. The *British Medical Journal*'s *How to do it*, now published in its second edition [8], contains brief chapters on all these aspects of research, originally written for medical readers but relevant to anyone in health care. Calnan's practical *Coping with research* [182] was written for medical beginners, and includes brief sections on speaking and writing. Smith's *Sources of information on remedial health* [1] contains a useful section on 'statistics, computing, experimental methods', which includes a further 22 references.

Partridge and Barnitt wrote *Research guidelines: a handbook for therapists* [184] after eight years of workshops and seminars, and the realization that there was nothing on the subject for therapists. It was written specifically for clinicians who want to undertake their own research, and contains a very useful wide-ranging glossary. Hawkins and Sorgi's *Research* [183] is a wide-ranging book which contains information on how to plan, speak and write about research. As well as a very good chapter by Jenkins on searching the literature, it has useful appendices on the MD thesis (useful for postgraduate paramedical theses), using a dictating machine, 'needless words causing verbosity' and American/British spelling.

When the research has been planned and carried out, figures may need to be correlated and probabilities calculated. Non-mathematicians will find Rowntree's *Statistics without tears* [189] a very helpful outline, with words and diagrams rather than formulae and equations. Other useful books for the beginner are Castle's

Statistics in small doses [186] and Petrie's *Lecture notes on medical statistics* [188], while more advanced statistics are contained in the *Essentials of medical statistics* by Kirkwood [187].

Writing up the results of research is a necessary step towards disseminating the information to a wider audience. Cormack's *Writing for nurses and allied professions* [194] is a basic book, containing practical exercises in each chapter and references for further reading. It covers writing in other fields too, as does *Professional writing for nurses* by Kolin and Kolin [196], although the clinical writing section may not be relevant for non-American writers.

Mitchell's *How to write reports* [197] is old now, but still very useful on report writing. *Thorne's Better medical writing* [198], now edited by S. Lock, is good for inexperienced writers writing for publication. It includes advice on what to do if your paper is rejected, and a list of words to avoid. The American Physical Therapy Association has published a collection of papers on writing (formerly published in *Physical Therapy*) as *Advice to authors* [190]. The Association has also published a *Style manual* [191] for writers for *Physical Therapy*, which covers writing abstracts and book reviews, and editorial style. Other allied health groups will find these useful.

Calnan has written two further practical books, on public speaking. *Speaking at medical meetings* [193] is aimed at the junior doctor who may have to speak at a meeting or conference, and contains clear basic advice. *How to speak and write* [192] covers a wider field and is aimed at nurses. Both are brief practical guides to the subject.

Reading other authors' papers can be helpful when creating a style of one's own, but their papers need careful assessment. Parry[7] has prepared some guidelines for appraising research papers in journals, including a list of 80 questions to ask. Having read many papers, some system of filing and indexing them is necessary, particularly for quick retrieval. Self[10] has compared six commercial software packages for computerizing such a system and considers the storage capacity required, ease of retrieval, ease of learning the system and so on. Roberts,[9] Mater[6] and Lehmkuhl[5] have all written on the organization of personal files, the first for medical readers and the others in physical therapy journals.

EDUCATION AND CAREERS

The *Directory of schools of medicine and nursing* [199] outlines qualifications and training in all branches of the health professions in the UK. It includes professions supplementary to medicine, professions related to medicine, alternative medicine professions and medical technicians. Detailed entries are given for each profession, as well as qualifications, registration and how to obtain both.

The American Medical Association's Committee on Allied Health Education and Accreditation (CAHEA) issues annually the *Allied Health Education Directory* [200], listing information on education for some allied health personnel. These include occupational therapists, nuclear medicine technologists, radiation therapy technologists and respiratory therapists. It lists accredited courses by specialty, subdivided by state and institution. CAHEA also distributes a bi-monthly *Newsletter* [201] containing, news, recent report summaries and a forthcoming events section. Volume 1 of Backus's *Medical and Health information directory* [152] contains information on US medical and allied health schools and colleges, but does not include speech therapy.

Clark's *Careers in nursing and allied professions* [202] contains brief information on allied health professions. Two short books on specific careers for allied health personnel are Ryckmans's *Working with disabled people* [203] and *Careers: working with the disabled* by Taylor [204].

MANAGEMENT AND ADMINISTRATION

Abstracts and indexes for health care management have been covered above, and articles on these subjects relating to allied health units and departments can be found using *Abstracts of Health Care Management Studies* [85], *Health Service Abstracts* [71], *HELMIS: Health Management Information Service* [87] or *Hospital Literature Index* [88]. Books on the management of allied health units and departments can be found using these and other bibliographies outlined above.

Statistical information for managers is explained by Day's *From facts to figures* [206], published by the King's Fund and giving easy practical advice. *Health and nursing management statistics* by Goldstone [207] is based on his lecture notes as Head of the School of Health Studies at Newscastle upon Tyne Polytechnic.

Computer software for managing departments, units or patient systems is regularly reviewed in professional journals. *British Journal of Healthcare Computing* publishes datafiles regularly, which list 'available computer systems in a particular healthcare application area'. The latest paramedical datafile was in 1987 [205] and listed 12 software applications in the paramedical fields covered in this volume, and a further 32 applications in other paramedical fields.

References

1. Brahmi, F. A. (1986). Verifying the elusive proceedings: a review of available sources. *Medical Reference Services Quarterly*, **5** (4), 1–11.
2. Callard, J. C. and Fruehauf, E. L. (1978). Comparison of American medical dictionaries. *Bulletin of the Medical Library Association*, **66** (3), 327–30.
3. Chamberlain, M. A. (1988). Disabled living centres. *British Medical Journal*, **296**, 1052–3.
4. Cochrane, C. G. and Mater, D. A. (1986). Selected information resources: infant health and development. *Physical and Occupational Therapy in Pediatrics*, **6** (3/4), 325–31.
5. Lehmkuhl, D. (1978). Techniques for locating, filing and retrieving scientific information. *Physical Therapy*, **58**, 579–84.

6. Mater, D. A. (1986). Managing your personal information files. *Physical and Occupational Therapy in Pediatrics*, **6**, 95–101.

7. Parry, A. (1987). Guide lines to appraising research papers in journals. *Physiotherapy*, **73** (7), 375–8.

8. Perry, C. A. (1985). HELMIS: a computerised database for health service management. In *Proceedings of the 8th International Online information meeting, London, 4–6 December 1984*. Oxford: Learned Information, pp. 365–72.

9. Roberts, D. C. (1984). The organization of personal index files. In Morton, L. T. and Godbolt, S. (eds), *Information sources in the medical sciences*. London: Butterworths, pp. 512–22.

10. Self, P. C. (1986). Creating personal index files. *Medical Reference Services Quarterly*, **5** (2), 15–26.

3 Current Awareness in the Paramedical Sciences

David Roberts

INTRODUCTION

As compared with that of core areas of medicine, which is of interest primarily to doctors, the information and research base of the paramedical or allied health professions is in general less well developed. While there is considerable variation between the various disciplines there now seems to be a movement towards improving the scientifically researched basis of allied health care. This is manifest in many ways, including increasing numbers of journal titles devoted primarily to these areas, of relevant professional articles and of meetings, conferences and post-qualification courses and associated activities. The problems of keeping up to date with all this growth are becoming more complex for allied health personnel.

This chapter will focus primarily on this question of continuing current awareness, although much of what is said about information sources and services will also be relevant to retrospective searching of the literature. The topics considered will be: mode, i.e. online, hardcopy etc.; some of the principal sources of information; types of published information, e.g. papers, articles, reports, news; and the criteria for making appropriate choices. The most important of these are coverage of the various sources and the cost of the searching activity.

MODE

By mode is meant the kind of information source consulted: personal communication, including courses, meetings and conferences; published sources (hard copy); and automated sources (online databases and compact disk, a relatively recent development in the provision of information services).

Personal Communication

Considerable reliance seems to be placed on personal communication, as Bohannon has noted in relation to physiotherapy.[3] In the correspondence sections of some journals, such as *Physiotherapy* [460] or the *British Journal of Occupational Therapy* [311], there are not infrequently requests for information related to a proposed project.

While personal communication may seem subjectively convincing and has the advantage of accessibility for most, it will to a considerable extent be subject to chance and opportunity. The information may be subjective or biased and will probably be incomplete. This kind of consideration may apply similarly to meetings and conferences and to courses, which may become dated, since they depend on considerable effort in preparation and update.

Published Sources

Published sources may range from small, irregular, local bulletins to the major bibliographies like *Index Medicus* [58] and *Excerpta Medica* [65]. Because of the preparation time required before the appearance of primary sources (journals) and the bibliographies citing them, these may not be as current as they seem. The *minimum* period for an article published in a British journal to be cited in *Index Medicus* is three months. In practice it may be longer. This must be added to the often lengthy period between completion of the research and publication of the article.

The major bibliographies will be a more comprehensive source of published information than personal communication. An indication of the numbers of citations in these sources is given below. However, none is fully comprehensive in any aspect of medicine. There are currently at least 10 000 journals published worldwide containing worthwhile articles pertaining to some aspect of medicine. *Index Medicus* includes about 3000 of these, from most of which most articles are taken. *Excerpta Medica* includes about 5000 but a greater number are selectively indexed (only selected articles are included). While there is considerable overlap between these sources, each includes titles not included by the other. It will be apparent that there is considerable material of potential relevance not included in either bibliography. This is particularly true of the allied health area.

Access to these major bibliographies may be limited by the high subscription costs. Only major institutions can afford them. Using them requires some knowledge and understanding of their indexing systems, a consideration that applies particularly to searching their online equivalents. A brief introduction to these indexing systems is given below.

Online Sources

The distinctive feature of online bibliographic databases, such as *Medline* [101] (*Index Medicus* online) and *EMBase* [100] (*Excerpta Medica* online) is their power and flexibility of searching. While hard copy modes allow only one access point for any enquiry (you can look up only one indexing term at a time), online searching permits the construction and entry of complex profiles combining indexing terms, authors and various other parameters. Effective searching requires knowledge not only of the indexing system but also of the searching software of the host system. A short section on some of the major host systems is included in this chapter.

Access to online systems may be inhibited not only by a lack of the necessary expertise in using them but also by the availability (or otherwise) of the necessary facilities – computer terminals, host and database passwords – at a convenient location.

Compact Disk (CD)

The application of compact disk technology to bibliographic databases is a relatively recent development. Such systems require access to a computer and a CD drive, as well as the necessary disks. With this equipment online running costs are eliminated.

At present there are several systems providing *Medline* on CD in the United Kingdom. All require some knowledge of the indexing system and of the searching methods of the particular system. These vary considerably and the results and output format that may be obtained also vary. In general, searching and output features are less flexible than in online searching. Only the Dialog system replicates online operations. A number of medical libraries in the United Kingdom have installed one of these systems.[10]

While other developments in information technology may have considerable potential to increase awareness in medicine, the applications that have been made do not impinge to any extent on the allied health area.

INFORMATION SOURCES

There are a large number of bibliographic databases having some relevance to medicine. Farbey has provided a comprehensive list with much relevant information [96]. Rossouw has recently reviewed information sources with reference to physiotherapists.[14] This review is also relevant to other specialities. Five specific information sources that will be of use to allied health professionals are now considered.

Index Medicus/Medline [58] and [101]

This database is produced by the National Library of Medicine in Bethesda, Maryland. The aim is international coverage of the whole of medicine although, as has already been noted, this is not comprehensive in the sense of including all possible journals of relevance. The journals selected are intended to reflect the research and practice in each country; probably these are the higher-quality journals. However, there seems to be some understandable bias towards American publications. There are about 5 500 000 records on the system dating from 1966. About 20 000 records are added to the system monthly.

Coverage of allied health areas is uneven. While there is a considerable amount of material relevant to, for example, physical therapy or speech therapy, coverage of these areas is far from comprehensive and coverage of some specialities, such as occupational therapy, is very sparse. Of the journals principally devoted to occupational therapy only the *American Journal of Occupational Therapy* [308] is included in *Index Medicus* and *Medline*. It is possible to qualify this statement because of the extensive range of interests of the occupational therapy profession. For example, those interested in psychiatric care will find material of relevance taken from the main psychiatric journals. There have been a number of recent studies of citation analyses in these areas.[1, 2, 7, 11] Comparison of the journal lists in these articles with the *List of Journals Indexed in Index Medicus* [56] or the more comprehensive *List of Serials Indexed for Online Users* [59] provides some confirmation of the selectivity of coverage.

The question of coverage is complex. If likely journal titles are known then a clue to the extent of coverage of the relevant literature may be obtained by looking for the title in the *List of Journals Indexed* [56]. In order to perform searches of *Index Medicus* or *Medline* efficiently it is necessary to have some knowledge of the indexing system. This is complex and comprehensive, aimed at maximizing retrieval power. A controlled thesaurus, *Medical Subject Headings (MeSH)*, of about 16 000 terms is used. *MeSH* appears in two forms, Public [60] and Annotated [61]. The latter is required for *Medline* and is certainly preferable for *Index Medicus*. It contains much extra information vital to effective indexing and searching. As well as being listed alphabetically in MeSH the terms are listed hierarchically in *Medical Subject Headings: Tree Structures (Trees)* [62].

This hierarchical arrangement provides a powerful retrieval tool as it is possible to enter a search statement so that the term itself and all those listed as more specific are searched. This, of course, applies only to online and some compact disk systems. In *Index Medicus* the headings are listed alphabetically, followed by details of the assigned citations.

Additional features of the indexing system are term definitions, term precoordination and the use of subheadings. Some terms are defined in special ways, a fact particularly applicable to health administration terms that are oriented to the US health care system. Only practice using the system and *Annotated MeSH* can help the user to understand how terms are used (although many are quite straight-forward). Many terms link concepts together; for example, 'liver' and 'disease' becomes 'liver diseases'. Indexers are instructed always to select the most specific term available, so the user may not find many citations on liver diseases under 'liver' or 'disease' and should not expect to find any on, for example, hepatitis (articles will be under 'hepatitis'). Assistance in identifying appropriate terms is provided by *Permuted Medical Subject Headings* [63], which lists the individual components of terms alphabetically, followed by a list of each term containing that component.

Further co-ordination is provided by the use of subheadings. These qualify or further define the meaning of headings – they indicate what aspect of the heading the article was about. An article on the drug treatment of Parkinsonism will be indexed 'Parkinson disease/drug therapy'. There are about 80 subheadings currently in use; the full list with brief definitions and rules concerning allowed heading/subheading combinations is included in *Annotated Mesh*. Most articles are listed in *Index Medicus* in two or three places corresponding to the main ideas of the article. Up to 12 more headings may be added for online searching.

This is no more than a brief introduction to *Index Medicus* and *Medline* although it is longer than the discussions of other systems that follow. More details may be found in *How to use Index Medicus and Excerpta Medica* by Strickland-Hodge [64], although he does not discuss in any depth the question of subject indexing. As the other sources considered here are broadly similar, less space is given to them, with the emphasis being on the differences.

Excerpta Medica/EMBase [65] and [100]

This database is produced by Elsevier Science Publishers. As noted above, some of the material included is in common with *Medline* and some different. The database is oriented to European and drug-related literature. It contains about 4 000 000 records dating from 1973 and about 25 000 records are added each month. The hard copy version is divided into a series of bibliographies corresponding to a variety of medical specialities. While many of these may contain material relevant to the allied health area the most relevant is probably the *Rehabilitation and Physical Medicine* series [476]. However, as with *Index Medicus* the coverage of the literature relevant to allied health seems to be selective and uneven. Again, an indication of the likely coverage of a specific enquiry may be obtained by comparing the *List of Journals Abstracted* [66] with known relevant journal titles.

Up to 1988 the indexing system for *EMBase* was based upon three controlled vocabularies and was radically different from and more complex than that of *Medline*. However, in 1988 a system very similar to that of *Medline* was introduced, although it differs in some details. As the principal interest here is current awareness a discussion of the earlier system is not included. Those who wish to conduct retrospective searches on *EMBase* should consult the *Guide to the classification and indexing system* [67] and Strickland-Hodge [64].

The principal user aid for the current system is the *Emtree classification* [68], which contains both alphabetic and hierarchical lists but does not have detailed annotations. Also available are lists of qualifiers (Drug links and Medical links), which are similar to the *MeSH* subheadings, and Emtags, which correspond to some very common concepts assigned to many articles. The structure and use of the thesaurus seem to be similar to those of *MeSH*; it may be anticipated that with increasing use and development the system will become more sophisticated with improved aids for the user.

Cumulated Index of Nursing and Allied Health (CINAHL) [69] and [97]

Produced by the CINAHL Corporation of Glendale, California, this database provides extensive coverage of nursing and allied health. The emphasis seems to be on nursing in all its aspects: the coverage of the allied health disciplines, although more extensive than that of *Medline*, still seems to be selective, especially with respect to some areas of interest to certain disciplines. Examples of such areas of relevance to allied health care are biomechanics and psychiatric rehabilitation. *CINAHL* is available online, in hard copy and as CD. It contains about 75 000 records from 1983 on and is updated bimonthly with about 3000 records.[5]

The indexing system is modelled very much on that of *Medline* in terms of the content and structure of the thesaurus and in the use of subheadings. Detailed additions and modifications have been made to accommodate the special requirements of the allied health disciplines,[6] but the methods of assignment of headings and co-ordination are very similar to those used for *Medline*.[8]

Entries in the list of indexing terms include annotations similar to but less detailed than MeSH [60]. The list also includes a guide to searching the database through three different host systems. A list of journals indexed is included in the bi-monthly issues of *CINAHL* and the list of indexing terms is also in the January/February issue each year.

DHSS-Data [99]

This is the online database of the Department of Health (formerly the Department of Health and Social Security) in London and is based on the library's abstracting and current awareness services. In terms of subject coverage the emphasis is on the administration and socio-economic aspects of health care and social welfare. As well as journal articles there are a large number of citations to different kinds of 'grey' literature, including pamphlets, reports and other official publications. As is well known, 'grey' literature is difficult to search and obtain so this is an invaluable source, at least with respect to the UK. The source materials are listed in the *Union list of periodicals currently received in headquarters libraries* [74]. *DHSS-Data* corresponds to a range of publications, including *Health Service Abstracts* [71], *Social Service Abstracts* [73] and *Nursing Research Abstracts* [72]. The database contains about

70 000 records from 1983 onwards and is updated weekly with about 1000 records per month.

As with the other information sources discussed there is a controlled thesaurus for indexing and searching [75]. This consists of about 22 000 entries, although about one-third of these refer the user to a preferred term. Useful features at each entry are scope notes and lists of broader, narrower and related terms and of synonyms.

Current Awareness Topics Services (CATS)

This is the most recently introduced of the services considered here. It is produced by the Medical Information Service of the British Library and is intended to provide comprehensive coverage of several of the allied health disciplines: complementary medicine, physiotherapy, occupational therapy, rehabilitation and terminal care. A monthly 'Index' publication is produced from the database for each of these areas [78]–[82]. Great emphasis is placed on comprehensiveness and currency – the maximum period between receipt of a journal and its appearance in one or more of the Index publications is one month (although this may be greater for certain items, for which *Medline* is used as a scanning tool). Roberts[12, 13] has described the origins of two of the publications. The total number of records is about 34 000, from early 1985 on, and is currently being increased at about 700 per month.

The indexing system in use is closely related to those of *Medline* and *CINAHL*. The basic vocabulary has been derived from MeSH but has been modified in accordance with the requirements of the subjects covered. An alphabetic list [83] containing scope notes and narrower and broader terms and a hierarchical list [84] are available. (These tools are only of use with the database.)

Although this system is not yet available online it is expected that it will be so in the near future. Retrospective and current awareness (monthly, quarterly, etc.) searches are available through the Medical Information Service at low cost. The aim has been to maximize availability with low subscriptions to the monthly Index publications. Registration with the British Library is not required for these services.

The Medical Information Service also produces a series of low-cost monthly bibliographies (Current Awareness Topics Searches) derived from *Medline*. Several of these are in the field of psychiatry, although the citations are frequently of a medical rather than rehabilitative nature. Two of these, *Hearing* [76] and *Language and Speech Disorders* [77], will be of interest to speech therapists.

More General Information

The discussion so far has been mainly of major bibliographic information services, mostly of the journal literature. There is, of course, a need for more general information concerning, for example, professional developments, political and social matters affecting health care and forthcoming meetings, courses and conferences, as well as reports and other more peripheral forms of information. In general, information provision of this kind is more decentralized and confusing than that of the journal literature. The System for Grey Literature in Europe (SIGLE) is an important resource but its coverage of health care may be selective and it may be difficult and expensive to obtain access.

As stated above, *DHSS-Data* covers at least some of this more general and special information but is oriented to the United Kingdom. The 'department' pages of many professional journals often contain news and details of meetings and courses pertaining to their speciality. Inspection of current issues may well be the most accessible source of such information. Some journals also include some form of bibliographic current awareness, although the comprehensiveness and currency of such services varies greatly. Journals with this kind of information include *Archives of Physical Medicine and Rehabilitation* [463], *International Journal of Rehabilitation Research* [45], *Journal of the American Dietetic Association* [599], *Journal of the American Podiatric Medical Association* [220], *Physiotherapy* [460] and *Physical Therapy* [465]. *Rehabilitation World* [51] contains a comprehensive list of international meetings and conferences impinging upon rehabilitation and related disciplines.

There are numerous information services produced locally giving both bibliographic and more general information. Mayhew[9] has recently argued the case for such services. Good examples of these are produced by the Disabled Living Foundation [156] and the National Demonstration Centre at Pinderfields Hospital, Wakefield, England [92]. Such services, although useful at the local level, tend to be limited in their coverage, not easily accessible or well known outside the local area and oriented to local (often relatively small) collections, usually those of the producing organization or library. (The extent to which these qualifying comments apply to specific services varies greatly; the two mentioned above seem to be less limited than many.)

Summary

Some general comments on the question of the subject coverage of the various information sources may be useful. The sources specializing in allied health care (*CATS* and *CINAHL*) do not in general include much material on chiropody, dietetics or radiography, although *CINAHL* does have material on radiographic technology. The more general sources, *Index Medicus* and *Excerpta Medica*, may be more useful for these specialities but, as was noted, their coverage will not be fully comprehensive. For occupational therapy, physiotherapy and complementary medicine, *CATS* may be the best source of recent references although it is as yet unavailable online. All aspects of the nursing literature that might contain information of relevance to allied health care are well covered by *CINAHL*. *DHSS-Data* is a useful resource for health administration and related matters within the United Kingdom and for grey literature.

The cost of using these resources will depend on the charges of the producer organization and of the host system (for online), and on the policy of the subscribing organization, who may charge their own users or offer the services without charge. If charges are made these may be for online time only or for full costs, including the use of a searching intermediary familiar with the system (often necessary). *Medline* is often found to be less expensive to use than other systems.

DATABASE HOSTS

Database hosts are companies that make a range of databases available as commercial operations. For medical databases three of the most important hosts are Dialog, Data-Star and Blaise-link (for National Library of Medicine databases). Some other hosts are listed by Farbey [96].

The choice of host will depend on several factors, including local accessibility, cost and range of databases offered. For the user the main consequence of this variety is the number of different types of searching software in use, that is, the methods of interrogating the computer. These vary considerably both in terms of the mechanics of operation and in the options of input and output of information. There is no space here to discuss these complexities but a useful summary of the different systems has been compiled by Arthur [95].

PHOTOCOPIES AND LOANS

Identification of articles of interest is the first stage of a bibliographic enquiry. Photocopies or, if appropriate, loans may be obtained in a variety of ways. The British Library Document Supply Centre (DSC) offers an international service based on its collections of about 120 000 journal titles. Of the 56 000 currently received titles about 10 000 are in the biomedical area. Access is through users registered with DSC. Because of recent increases in the price of photocopy forms some users may wish to restrict their own organizations' use of the DSC service. University, medical and many hospital libraries have their own large collections, although these are less comprehensive than that of the DSC. These may be a less expensive source of photocopies than the DSC, depending on the policy of the library concerned. Many libraries participate in more or less formal inter-library services in order to make available a wider range of materials than their own collections. NHS libraries have links of this kind, which bypass the centralized service based on DSC and provide originals and photocopies at a lower cost. For those without access to either of these sources the British Library Medical Information Service provides a service not requiring registration. However, this is limited to photocopies from stock only (no inter-library search), may be relatively slow (several days) and costs the same as the main service for registered users.

Bohannon, a prolific author on, among other things, aspects of the literature for physical therapists, recently suggested that departments should take an active role in circulating photocopies to members of staff.[4]

CONCLUSIONS

This review of information sources and services in the allied health area shows that there is a considerable range at varying cost. The choice to be made will depend upon the subject matter and the finance available as well as on the practical matter of accessibility. As none of the sources is fully comprehensive it is preferable to avoid reliance on any single one.[3] There seems to be a powerful case for combining at least some of the resources employed in providing the plethora of information sources, to create a single, comprehensive service for allied health professionals. No such project is on the horizon, so users are faced with difficult choices in their information requirements and in particular in current awareness.

References

1. Bohannon, R. W. (1986). Citation analysis of *Physical Therapy*: a special communication. *Physical Therapy*, **66** (4), 540-1.
2. Bohannon, R. W. (1987). Core journals of physiotherapy. *Physiotherapy Practice*, **3** (3), 126-8.
3. Bohannon, R. W. (1988). How to find relevant references for a publication. *Physiotherapy Practice*, **4** (1), 41-4.
4. Bohannon, R. W. and Larking, P. A. (1986). Current journal article provision for the physical therapy clinicians of one department. *Physical Therapy*, **66** (5), 689-90.
5. Fishel, C. C. (1985). The Nursing and Allied Health (*CINAHL*) database: a guide to effective searching. *Medical Reference Services Quarterly*, **4** (3), 1-16.
6. Fishel, C. C. (1985). *CINAHL* list of subject headings: a nursing thesaurus revised. *Bulletin of the Medical Library Association*, **73** (2), 153-9.
7. Johnson, K. S. and Leising, D. J. (1985). The literature of occupational therapy. A citation analysis study. *American Journal of Occupational Therapy*, **40** (6), 390-6.
8. Lansing, P. S. and Edmondson, M. E. (1987). Subject indexing of the *American Journal of Occupational Therapy* in *Medline* and *NAHL*. *Medical Reference Services Quarterly*, **6** (2), 39-49.
9. Mayhew, J. (1988). A case for local current-awareness publications. *Health Libraries Review*, **5** (1), 61-5.
10. Pentelow, G. M. (1989). New technology in medical libraries. *British Medical Journal*, **298** (6678), 907-8.
11. Reed, K. L. (1988). Occupational therapy articles in serial publications. *Bulletin of the Medical Library Association*, **76** (2), 125-30.
12. Roberts, D. J. (1986). *CATS*: a new information service in physiotherapy. *Physiotherapy*, **72** (11), 533-5.

13. Roberts, D. J. (1988). A new information service for occupational therapists. *British Journal of Occupational Therapy*, **51** (10), 353–4.
14. Rossouw, S. F. (1986). Information sources in physiotherapy. *South African Journal of Physiotherapy*, **42** (1), 5–9.

4 Chiropody

Erica South

J. C. Dagnall, the leading living authority on the history of the chiropody profession, said in 1965[1] that a professional group can be judged not only by the state of its libraries but also by the literature it has produced. It follows that chiropody, as a profession of comparatively recent origin, and with its subject matter confined within relatively narrow limits, has not produced vast quantities of literature.

Members of the profession are now, increasingly, demanding information for various reasons. In the UK first degree courses have been instituted: the schools of chiropody are contemplating the transition from a three-year diploma course to that of a first degree course. Chiropodists who have a first degree are embarking on postgraduate qualifications. There is great pressure on all professionals to pursue continuing education and self-development. Chiropodists have become aware that to be taken seriously as a profession they must undertake and publish properly validated research.

NOMENCLATURE

At this stage, it might be as well to explain the difference between the terms 'chiropody' and 'podiatry'. First it must be admitted that etymologically 'podiatry' is the more accurate term; 'chiropody' is a hybrid term that means 'hand and foot', and is thus, pedantically speaking, misleading. There is, however, no difference between the two terms. The term podiatry is exclusively used in the USA, and was introduced to emphasize the difference between fully trained practitioners and those who had merely undertaken a correspondence or other short course. It has been fairly successful in the USA and the public are probably more aware of the difference. British chiropodists are now thinking along the same lines.

The qualification gained by the three-year full-time course in the UK is to be called the Diploma in Podiatric Medicine from 1989, and one school, the London Foot Hospital and School of Chiropody, has become the London Foot Hospital and School of Podiatric Medicine. American podiatrists follow a four-year course full-time and are qualified to undertake day surgery on completion. In the UK, the full-time three-year course entitles students to exemption from sections 1 to 4 of the Surgical course of the Society of Chiropodists; they must complete section 5 with an examination and then undertake section 6 (which involves operating under supervision) before they are considered competent to perform ambulatory foot surgery.

HISTORY OF THE PROFESSION

Like all members of the medical professions, the chiropodist began in a lowly position. The first practitioners were street vendors of their skills. Ben Jonson includes a corn cutter with his street cry among the *dramatis personae* of *Bartholomew Fair*, first staged in 1614. Towards the end of the seventeenth century the corn cutters were advertising in the newspapers and shops and practising in the coffee houses and bathhouses of the time; they were no longer street traders. In the eighteenth century they printed trade cards and practised from their own premises. It should also be noted that they advertised their skills as both dentists and chiropodists – a common practice on the Continent at that time.

The term 'chiropodist' was first used by David Low,[6] who had translated into English a French book on chiropody written by a surgeon who specialized in chiropody, N.-L. La Forêt.[3] The first original book on chiropody in the English language was published by Heyman Lion.[5] Lion must also be remembered because he was the first practitioner to realize that a knowledge of medicine and surgery would be useful, and he studied both subjects at Edinburgh University.

The next landmark was the publication of Lewis Durlacher's book.[2] Durlacher was the first to conceive the idea of forming an association of chiropodists and, although this did not occur in his lifetime, his nephew was to be involved in the initial discussions which eventually led to the formation of the first British society. He later withdrew from any active part in the body thus formed. The National Society of Chiropodists was formed in 1913 by a group of practising chiropodists and interested doctors. The Society of Chiropodists is the direct descendant of the National Society.

Durlacher's book was also published in America during the same year, 1845, and was the first chiropodial book to appear there. The first original work by an American chiropodist was a small treatise published by George A. White in 1869.[10] Twenty-six years later (and, it must be noted, before the formation of a

British society) the Pedic Society of New York was founded. This society started the journal *Pedic Items* in 1907, which later became the *Journal of the American Podiatric Medical Association* [220], the foremost podiatric journal in the USA to this day.

PERIODICALS

Chiropody

The most recent information is always found in periodicals, and while there are not many specifically directed to chiropodists there are several that are of great interest and particular relevance. The only British journal of any significance in the field is *The Chiropodist* [214], published monthly by the Society of Chiropodists, now in A4 format and improving. Unfortunately it is not indexed by any of the indexing databases, and one is forced to rely on the annual index published in the journal. This is not professionally produced and it can be difficult to find a specific reference.

The American Podiatric Medical Association also publishes a monthly journal, *The Journal of the American Podiatric Medical Association* [220]. This is indexed by *Index Medicus* [58]. It also contains a *Bibliography of Podiatric Medicine and Surgery* compiled with the assistance of the National Library of Medicine.

There is one other serial specifically directed towards chiropodists that should not be ignored. This is *Clinics in Podiatric Medicine and Surgery* [218], which was first issued in 1984 and appears quarterly. Each issue is devoted to one subject, in the style of the other *Clinics* series, and articles are both comprehensive and well researched. Each issue contains a cumulated index for the current year. This journal is also indexed in *Index Medicus*.

Related Subjects

There are several journals in fields of interest to chiropodists, but which are not directed specifically towards them. In the area of orthopaedics the *Journal of Foot Surgery* [224] is published monthly by the American College of Foot Surgeons and started publication in 1961. *Foot and Ankle* [219] is published by the American Orthopaedics Foot and Ankle Society and is a bi-monthly which first appeared in 1980. Also of interest are the *Journal of Bone and Joint Surgery*, which has two series, the American series [222] having nine issues and the British series [223] five issues a year; this journal started in 1903. *Clinical Orthopaedics and Related Research* [217], which was first published in 1951, is a monthly and often has material of interest to chiropodists.

Chiropodists are becoming increasingly involved with sports medicine and both the *British Journal of Sports Medicine* [212], published four times a year by the British

Association of Sport and Medicine, and the *American Journal of Sports Medicine* [209] contain material of interest.

Closely related to orthopaedics is the study of biomechanics, and here there are several journals, two of which chiropodists will find useful. *Journal of Biomechanics* [221] appears monthly, and *Clinical Biomechanics* [216], which is sponsored by the Osteopathic Association, is a quarterly journal that started publication in 1985.

Among the many diabetic journals, *Practical Diabetes* [225], which is published bi-monthly, is recommended. Other periodicals that would prove interesting and useful are listed in Part II [208]–[226].

CURRENT AWARENESS SERVICES AND ABSTRACTS

Bibliography of Podiatric Medicine and Surgery is a monthly current awareness listing on chiropody, which appears in *Journal of the American Podiatric Medical Association* [220]. It covers the periodicals indexed in *Index Medicus* and is arranged by the same *MeSH* headings.

At the time of writing (June 1989) the British Library Medical Information Service has not produced a monthly current awareness bulletin specifically aimed at chiropodists, which must surely come in the future. However, at present there are three indexing services that are of interest. The first is *RECAL: Rehabilitation Engineering Current Awareness Listings* [228] from the National Centre for Training and Education in Prosthetics and Orthotics, which appears twice a month. This carries listings from journals taken by the Centre itself.

Next is *Sports Medicine Bulletin* [229], which is a monthly listing of articles on all aspects of sports medicine from a wide range of journals, published by the London Sports Medical Institute and the British Library Medical Information Service. There is also the quarterly *Diabetes Contents* [227], which reproduces the contents pages of all leading English language diabetic journals, and contains citations of papers on diabetes from leading non-diabetic journals in which such papers appear frequently. This is published by the British Diabetic Association.

Finally the South West Thames Regional Library Service produces a brief monthly sheet called *What to Read – Feet* [230], which is distributed widely and can be obtained either from an NHS librarian or via the local regional librarian.

The only abstracting service is that published annually in hardback format by Year Book Medical Publishers and edited by Richard Jay, *The Year Book of Podiatric Medicine and Surgery* [231]. It has appeared annually since 1985 and has abstracts of interest to podiatrists and chiropodists culled from over 500 journals in the English language. The abstracts are arranged by subject chapters and it has a good index. The title has the date of the current year as a prefix.

BOOKS

Development of the Literature

J. C. Dagnall[1] and Walter Seelig,[8] both of whom are extremely interested in the history of chiropody, have written detailed articles in *The Chiropodist* tracing the early history of chiropodial writing.

Very few books on chiropody were published in the UK or USA before this century. The first book on chiropody to appear in the UK was *Chiropodologia* by Low,[6] which was mentioned above. The most important work on chiropody to be published in the UK during the nineteenth century was Durlacher's *Treatise on corns, bunions, the diseases of the nails and the general management of the feet*,[2] also mentioned above. This book is surprisingly relevant even now.

The next milestone was the publication of Wagner's *Handbook of chiropody*,[9] which was illustrated with photographs. This was followed by Lewi's *Textbook of chiropody*,[4] the first textbook for students, which was published in the USA but contained a chapter by E. G. V. Runting. Runting was an English chiropodist involved with the foundation of the National Society of Chiropodists; he wrote a book that was intended to be a training manual for army chiropodists. This was followed, after the First World War, by his *Practical chiropody*.[7]

The Foot

During the 1930s two books were published on the structure of the foot that are still considered to be important source materials. One was *The foot* [260] by Norman Lake, a physician who lectured at the London Foot Hospital, which had been founded by the National Society of Chiropodists. The other was *The human foot* [269] by an American orthopaedic surgeon, D. J. Morton. Later came another classic on the structure of the human foot by F. Wood Jones [257], a lecturer in anatomy at the University of Manchester.

There are two books, both recently published, that cover all or most aspects of the foot in a comprehensive way. The first is *The foot* [251]; this is an excellent work and has numerous reference from both sides of the Atlantic. The other, Regnaud's *The foot* [275], is translated from the French, the author being a surgeon who specializes in the foot; he covers many aspects of the foot but specifically writes to set out his own methods of treatment.

There are two anatomical atlases that deserve mention. The first is in the well-known series of colour atlases from Wolfe Medical Publications, the *Colour atlas of foot and ankle anatomy* [265] by R. M. H. McMinn; the author is an expert in this field and the book is well-produced and inexpensive. The other is the *Atlas of podiatric anatomy* by Mercado [267], which has beautifully prepared overlying plates and is a delight to use.

Biomechanics

Chiropodists are becoming increasingly involved in biomechanics and sports medicine. In the former subject there is no doubt that the two-volume *Clinical biomechanics* by Root *et al.* [276] is a classic text. It is, however, quite expensive and there is a new edition in preparation. The other volume that should be mentioned is the *Compendium of podiatric biomechanics* edited by Sgarlato [281], which is out of print. Pressure may be exerted on the California College of Podiatric Medicine (which published it) for a copy. An important survey was made of the feet of recruits to the Canadian army in 1947 by R. H. Harris [250] and this is frequently quoted in the literature. About 20 years later the American Academy of Orthopaedic Surgeons published *Joint motion* [233], which is still used as a reference work today. Inman's book *Human walking* [254] is essential reading in this field, and we should not overlook Ducroquet's *Walking and limping* [245]. Specific books on sports medicine are not mentioned here as there are so many and none of them is written by or for chiropodists.

Orthotics

Charlesworth, a chiropodist, wrote *Chiropodial orthopaedics* [239] and thereby coined a term for what is now called orthotics or appliance-making. This was the first book written for chiropodists on this subject, and although there are many new materials and methods, it is still relevant in some respects today. The most recent book in this field is *Practical orthotics for chiropodists* [243] by Coates, a lecturer at the Chelsea School of Chiropody. For those who require greater scientific insight, there is a section on feet in the *Atlas of orthotics* [232], sponsored by the American Academy of Orthopaedic Surgeons.

Radiology of the foot is still comparatively new as a diagnostic tool. A recent issue of *Clinics in Podiatric Medicine and Surgery* [242] gives an extremely comprehensive review of the present state of the discipline. Weissman's *Radiology of the foot* [287] is the most comprehensive work on the subject. There is also a good chapter in *The foot* [251] by a radiographer and a radiologist.

Foot Surgery

Many books relevant to chiropodists are written by orthopaedic surgeons, and those on surgery of the foot are all in that category and all also by Americans. Possibly the foremost in this field is *Fundamentals of foot surgery*, edited by E. D. McGlamry [264], which is a major contribution to podiatric literature, with many illustrations, tables and charts. The material is without exception well referenced. *Surgery of the foot*, by K. K. Wu [289], has good chapters on foot and ankle trauma although there is not very much on biomechanics, which detracts from its usefulness. Mann's *Surgery of the foot* [266], although authoritative and comprehensive, lacks much of specific relevance for chiropodists, which is regrettable.

There is only one comprehensive text on therapeutics, *Yale's Podiatric medicine* [291], which is profusely illustrated and well referenced. The original author was an American podiatrist and the work has recently been revised by his son, also a podiatrist.

Paediatric and Geriatric Podiatry

There is one outstanding book on podopaediatrics written by a podiatrist, Tax [283], which provides sound, scientific and time-tested information. One other, *The child's foot* by Tachdjian [282], should be mentioned. This was written by a paediatric orthopaedic surgeon and, while it is extremely authoritative, it contains much material outside the scope of chiropody.

There is little written on the geriatric foot. However, many books on the general care of the elderly contain a chapter on foot care; the speciality is also covered in the literature on the rheumatoid foot and the diabetic foot. The January 1988 issue of *Clinics in Podiatric Medicine and Surgery* [241] on the rheumatoid foot contains useful articles and recent references from both the UK and the USA. The collected reports from the Arthritis and Rheumatism Council [234] should not be forgotten. *Clinics in Podiatric Medicine and Surgery* also devoted a recent issue [240] to the diabetic foot, which is extremely useful, and the papers of a British symposium on the foot in diabetes have been published [244]. Another good text on this controversial subject is the recent *Management of the diabetic foot* by Brennan [238]. Finally there is Baran and Dawber's unique book, *Diseases of the nails* [236]. This is a classic, well-illustrated, well-written and with plenty of current references.

There are several books on the skin that are of interest. Only one was written specifically for chiropodists, *Podiatric dermatology* [263], which covers the subject comprehensively. Jarrett's nine-volume work on the skin [256], which covers every aspect of the physiology and pathology of the skin and hair, is also recommended.

REPORTS

The majority of reports and surveys that have been published in the UK have been carried out by practising chiropodists and published in *The Chiropodist*. There is a useful checklist in *The Chiropodist* [299] of surveys published in this journal between 1945 and 1969. Surveys published since 1970 will have to be traced by keyword or subject matter in the indexes of *The Chiropodist*.

During the past decade surveys have been published by researchers outside the profession. In 1983, Kemp and Winkler published a major sociological survey [297] directly related to chiropody. They had examined the National Health Service Chiropody Service and pointed to ways in which it could be modified for the benefit of both patients and practitioners to make it more efficient and more cost-effective.

In 1985 the DHSS commissioned Ann Cartwright and Gregor Henderson to look at the unmet needs of elderly people for chiropody services. Their report [294] concluded that the service would need to be doubled, but that it would be cost-effective to do so. A survey made in 1969 by Clarke [296] found that, as people got older, more things went wrong with their feet. Very recently a survey was undertaken by chiropodists in Wessex [293], who wanted to establish the foot health levels of the population at different ages. This was carried out during 1982–85 and over 700 people were interviewed.

Two national reports have been carried out investigating the consequences of badly fitting shoes for children, and issued by the Chancellor of the Exchequer [295] and the National Consumer Council [298]. Both the Shoe and Allied Trades Research Association (SATRA) [1128] and C. and J. Clark [1269] have carried out surveys and research on matters relevant to chiropodists and can be contacted; it should be noted that some of the SATRA reports are confidential.

LIBRARIES

The Society of Chiropodists has archival material related to the profession (see below) and offers advice on professional matters, but there is no collection of current materials for chiropodists to consult. Other libraries that may prove useful are those of the 16 schools of chiropody. These vary in content as some have been better funded in the past than others, but all can provide some help, since they belong to a loose inter-school network and can draw on the resources of other schools. NHS district libraries, postgraduate medical centres and colleges of nursing may provide reference facilities to health care professionals (although some do not), and some will grant full library and information facilities. The British Medical Association (BMA) has a system of institutional membership that gives full use of its library; it is worth finding out whether use can be made of this large medical library. Those who are pursuing some form of education, whether basic, postbasic or postgraduate, will have access to the library of the institution to which they are attached. The librarians will be able to offer help and advice in obtaining material.

Historical Collections

The Society of Chiropodists [1043], the direct descendant of the National Society, holds archive material relating to the profession. It also has a library that possesses books of historical interest relating to the profession. The society plans to make this material much easier to consult in the near future, but meanwhile it is possible to arrange to refer to it (although it is not yet properly catalogued). Various eminent chiropodists have left their collections of early chiropodial writings to the society during the past. The society is also a trade union and has a collection of papers relating to industrial relations in the profession, and evidence given to the Pay Review Body.

The Center for the History of Footcare and Footwear [1279] was formed at the Pennsylvania College of Podiatric Medicine in 1981 by the amalgamation of the libraries of two well-known American podiatrists who were particularly interested in the history of their profession. An occasional bulletin is issued by the curator.

The Central Museum at Northampton [1256], the British centre for the shoe trade, has a large collection of shoes, lasts etc., and an extremely knowledgeable curator. C. and J. Clark began making shoes over 150 years ago, and have a museum at Street in Somerset of shoes worn in Britain since Roman and medieval times [1269]. They also have early shoemaking machinery and a collection of cartoons concerning shoes and shoemakers. They maintain archives and have many documents relating to the history of the firm and to shoemaking.

William Footman set up the Footman Collection [1243] in memory of his father, who had founded the family chiropodial supplies firm in 1948. This museum contains equipment, appliances and books from all over the UK that pertain to chiropody. It also has journals, trade catalogues, invoices and account books, foot appliances and shoe lasts. There is an extensive collection of all kinds and exhibits are constantly being added. It is now being catalogued by the Wellcome Museum for the History of Medicine, which is in itself part of the Science Museum.

ORGANIZATIONS

The Shoe and Allied Trades Research Association (SATRA) [1128] is a long-established organization that has sponsored much useful research. It publishes a monthly *Bulletin* [226], which contains research reports and progress on current projects. It also publishes fashion digests and technological studies.

The Foot Health Council [1125] sponsors an annual Foot Health Week, which takes place in May. It publishes leaflets and brochures on foot health education, and has made several videos on foot health for specific groups of the population. The council also publishes the *Children's Foot Health Register* [213] each year, which informs shoppers who wish to have trained advice in fitting children's shoes.

References
1. Dagnall, J. C. (1965). The history of chiropodial literature. *The Chiropodist*, **20** (7), 173–84.
2. Durlacher, L. (1845). *Treatise on corns, bunions, the diseases of the nails and general management of the feet*. London: Simpkin Marshall.
3. La Forêt, N.-L. (1781). *L'art de soigner les pieds, contenant un traité sur les cors, verrues, durillons, oignons, engelures, les accidens des ongles et leur difformités*. Paris: F. J. Desoer.

4. Lewi, M. J. (1914). *The textbook of chiropody*. New York: The School of Chiropody.

5. Lion, H. (1802). *An entire new and original work being a complete treatise upon spinae pedum*. Edinburgh: H. Inglis.

6. Low, D. (1785). *Chiropodologia, or, a scientific enquiry into the causes of corns, warts, onions and other painful or offensive cutaneous excrescences*. London: J. Rozea.

7. Runting, E. G. V. (1925). *Practical chiropody*. London: London Scientific Press.

8. Seelig, W. (1953). Studies in the history of chiropody. *The Chiropodist*, **8** (8), 381–97.

9. Wagner, F. (1903). *A handbook of chiropody*. London: Osborne, Garrett.

10. White, G. A. (1869). *A practical monograph on the treatment of local complaints of the feet*. Washington: Pearson.

5 Occupational Therapy
Margie Mellis

INTRODUCTION

Occupational therapy is a developing profession, one of the paramedical services that is concerned with improving the quality of life of the mentally and physically ill and disabled. Treatment is by the use of activities, carefully selected by the therapist, to help patients achieve their highest level of physical, mental and social independence. The patient's participation and co-operation are of the greatest importance, and therefore the occupational therapist needs to find the most stimulating and appropriate activity for each individual's needs.

The aim is to help the person practise all the activities involved in self-care, work and leisure. Activities are used to strengthen muscles, increase movement and restore co-ordination and balance. With people who are mentally ill similar activities are used to provide structure, support and the development of skills and self-confidence. Where someone has a lasting impairment or disability occupational therapists will teach special ways of doing everyday things and may also provide various aids and equipment if these are needed.

Occupational therapists are trained to assess patients and to plan courses of treatment that are individually tailored to the needs of each patient. As the needs of the patient change so will the treatment, and occupational therapists work closely with patients and their families. They are often called upon to give emotional support and counselling to help people come to terms with illness or disability.

Occupational therapists are involved in many different fields, with people who are physically disabled or mentally ill, with people who are mentally handicapped, with children and the elderly. In the UK they work within the National Health Service, in local authority social services, in private practice, in special schools and in voluntary organizations.

HISTORY AND DEVELOPMENT OF THE PROFESSION

Occupational therapy is a fairly recent discipline compared to others in the medical and social fields, although Macdonald[14] and Hopkins[12] demonstrate that the healing properties of work, exercise and play on which occupational therapy is based were recognized and utilized thousands of years ago and have continued to be appreciated since then.

The term 'occupational therapy' originated in 1914, when George Barton, a founder member of the society that became the American Occupational Therapy Association, suggested that it was the term that, taken in its fullest sense, best described the service offered. Under that name, occupational therapy was first introduced into Britain in 1919 by Dr Henderson at the Glasgow Royal Mental Hospital, Gartnavel. The beneficial effects of occupation, however, particularly in the treatment of mental patients, had long been apparent and the occupational therapist of today gradually came into being as an important member of the paramedical team. Macdonald points out that occupational therapy emerged 'by a process of evolution and experiment'.[14]

Initially, occupational therapy was used in the mental hospitals. During the French Revolution, in 1786, Philippe Pinel introduced 'prescribed physical exercises and manual occupations' as a method of treatment in the Bicêtre Asylum for the Insane near Paris. He asserted that 'the return of convalescent patients to their previous interests, to the practice of their profession, to industriousness and perseverance have always been for me the best omen of final recovery'.[17] This is not only the first reference in the literature to medically prescribed use of work for remedial purposes, but is also still a central part of the philosophy of occupational therapy.

The use of work therapy continued to flourish in the mental hospitals of Europe and North America throughout the nineteenth century, but it was not until the end of that century that occupational therapy began to be applied to physical as well as mental conditions. For example, in 1890 Dr Philip of Edinburgh questioned the value of continued rest in the treatment of tuberculosis and advocated instead carefully prescribed activities and exercise. It was not until the First World War, however, that the value of occupational therapy in the treatment of physical conditions was clearly demonstrated. Canada was the first country to set up a programme of occupational therapy, and when the USA came into the war they borrowed a Canadian, T. B. Kidner, to organize the work in their military hospitals.

In Britain, Sir Robert Jones, the eminent surgeon, persuaded the War Office to set up orthopaedic centres. The success of his centre at Shepherd's Bush in

London and the setting up of training schools at Bristol and Edinburgh in the 1930s encouraged the Ministry of Health to establish rehabilitation workshops during the Second World War.

The history and development of occupational therapy throughout the world is well documented by Licht[13] and Mendez,[15] while Hopkins[12] gives a detailed picture of the situation in North America and Macdonald[14] concentrates on the development in England. Zara Groundes-Peace[10] covers the history of occupational therapy in Scotland and the situation in Canada is well covered in a commemorative issue of the *Canadian Journal of Occupational Therapy*.[4] All these sources have excellent bibliographies for those who are particularly interested in the history of the profession and wish to explore it in more detail. Anyone who would like to read early contemporary texts on occupational therapy will find a list in Reed and Sanderson [401].

PROFESSIONAL BODIES

The first professional association to be founded, in 1917, was the United States' National Society for the Promotion of Occupational Therapy. This was changed in 1923 to its present title, the American Occupational Therapy Association. Margaret Fulton, who had qualified in the USA, became the first trained occupational therapist to be employed in a British hospital when she was appointed to the Royal Mental Hospital in Aberdeen in 1925; in 1932 she and several other occupational therapists became aware of the need for a professional association and the Scottish Association of Occupational Therapists was formed with 11 members. It was disbanded during the Second World War and reconstituted in 1946. The Association of Occupational Therapists was formed in England in 1936 and the two associations became united as the British Association of Occupational Therapists in 1974. This remains the only professional association for occupational therapists in the United Kingdom. Its functions, as stated in the *Occupational therapists' reference book* [347], are 'to set standards for entry into the profession; and for performance and behaviour of members admitted to the profession; to foster development and research into the work of the profession; and to represent the views of the profession'.

In 1978 the British Association of Occupational Therapists became an independent trade union and the College of Occupational Therapists [1056] was formed to cater for the professional and educational aspects of the association's work. In 1989 the college's headquarters moved from Rede Place in London to a new information and study centre in Marshalsea Road. The need for a new centre reflects the growth of the profession and the demands made on occupational therapists to evaluate the latest techniques and to offer an effective service. The centre has conference and seminar facilities, provides a meeting place for disabled people and their carers, and it is intended that a resource centre will be developed.

The British Association of Occupational Therapists and the College of

Occupational Therapists publish many books and leaflets on all aspects of occupational therapy, including the biennial *Occupational therapists' reference book* [347], which is an invaluable reference tool with a fund of information about the profession, special-interest groups and treatment media for the many different fields in which occupational therapists are involved. The sections on treatment media are particularly useful for their extensive bibliographies and lists of contact groups. As well as these bibliographies at the end of each section, there are several pages of sources of reference at the end of the book, which form in effect an up-to-date bibliography of occupational therapy.

The United Kingdom is a member country of the World Federation of Occupational Therapists [1016]. Set up in 1952 with representatives from six countries to promote the development of occupational therapy and to safeguard professional standards, it has continued to grow so that today there are 35 member countries. Delegates from these countries meet every two years to conduct the business of the federation and a congress is held every four years at which there is an opportunity to present both clinical and research papers specifically related to occupational therapy. Proceedings are published and give details of research papers [419].

EDUCATION AND TRAINING

The professional training of occupational therapists in the UK began in 1930 when Dr Elizabeth Casson set up the Dorset House School of Occupational Therapy at her psychiatric clinic in Bristol; this school is now at Oxford. In Scotland, the Astley Ainslie Occupational Therapy Training Centre was set up at Edinburgh in 1936. There are now 24 courses in the UK, both full-time and part-time: 18 in England, three in Scotland, two in Wales and one in Northern Ireland. Most schools offer a three-year course leading to the award of the Diploma of the College of Occupational Therapists, but three schools now offer a degree course (a three-year degree course at Queen Margaret College in Edinburgh, a four-year honours degree course at the University of Ulster at Jordanstown, and an extra year on top of the three-year diploma course at Christchurch College in Canterbury), and many more are in the process of implementing a degree course. The Essex School of Occupational Therapy has a two-year accelerated course for suitably qualified graduates, as does the School of Occupational Therapy at the London Hospital Medical College, and six centres offer a four-year in-service course for occupational therapy helpers. A list of the schools can be found in Alexander [199].

The education and training of occupational therapists is carefully monitored and validated by the Occupational Therapists Board of the Council for Professions Supplementary to Medicine (CPSM). CPSM is a statutory body set up under the Professions Supplementary to Medicine Act of 1960 with a remit covering seven specific professions, each represented by a board. As a completely independent body it regulates education and training and controls the quality of that training and of the professional qualifications granted. Registration with CPSM is thus an indication that an individual has achieved certain educational and clinical standards, and without state registration a qualified occupational therapist cannot practise in the National Health Service or local authority social services. According to CPSM's annual report there were 10 665 registered occupational therapists in 1989.

Until the early 1980s the occupational therapy course had not undergone many changes. However, as a result of a working party established by the College of Occupational Therapists and the Occupational Therapy Board of the Council for Professions Supplementary to Medicine, a report, *Diploma course 1981* [430], was published to take account of modern educational knowledge and trends. All UK schools now implement this course. The occupational therapist's course includes the principles and practice of occupational therapy, anatomy, physiology, psychology, sociology, medical and surgical conditions, and psychiatry, as well as techniques and skills used in treatment and research, administration and management. The course generally lasts three years and includes practice placements in a wide variety of clinical situations.

In 1987 the Manpower Planning Advisory Group commissioned the National Health Service Training Authority to examine and plan the future staffing and training and education arrangements for occupational therapy services provided by the social services and the national health service. The report of this committee, chaired by Dr Peter Horrocks, is expected in 1990. The committee worked closely with an Independent Commission, chaired by Louis Blom-Cooper, which was set up at the same time by the College of Occupational Therapists to review the demands on the resources available to the profession up to the year 2010. It subsequently broadened its remit to look at all aspects of the profession, present and future, and to make recommendations on the way forward [439a].

One of the recommendations made by the Commission was that occupational therapists should prepare for an increased role in community care. Occupational therapists have in fact been community based for many years. Their role in social services departments developed largely as a response to the statutory obligations placed on local authorities by the Chronically Sick and Disabled Persons Act 1970 to provide certain services for people registered as chronically sick or disabled. This initially involved the prescription and provision of disability equipment and the assessment and recommendation of adaptations to the person's home. However, this role has developed and the occupational therapist working with people in the community has become 'more of an enabler, aimed at helping the disabled person to maximize his independence and quality of life'.[11]

The UK government's policy on care in the community, with its emphasis on resettlement and integration, has meant that there is an increased demand for the services of the occupational therapist. The value of this service was recognized in a debate on occupational therapy services in the House of Commons in July 1989, when the Parliamentary Under-Secretary of State for Health, Mr Roger

Freeman, stated that 'occupational therapists are often the key to the continued independence of the many people who are now rightly living in the community rather than in the various forms of institutional care'.[11]

The Independent Commission under Blom-Cooper further recognized that there was a shortage of trained occupational therapists and recommended that an 80 per cent increase in numbers would be necessary to support the proposed expansion. There are now 10 665 state-registered occupational therapists, and 930 students commenced training in 1988. This number has been increasing annually and extra places are being funded. Several new schools have opened recently and student intake has increased. The Commission believes that, despite the urgent need for more occupational therapists, the profession should not vary its standards of entry for training and that the move towards degree status is to be encouraged.

The move towards a degree is seen as a natural progression as the profession develops and expands. Occupational therapy is one of the fastest-growing paramedical professions and the body of knowledge that forms the theoretical basis for the practice of occupational therapy has grown in complexity to such an extent that the qualified occupational therapist requires more than the current diploma course can offer. In particular there is an increasing emphasis on the importance of research, on introducing occupational therapy students to a lifelong commitment to questioning and evaluation. 'Occupational therapy education', according to Mary Green, 'is at the beginning of a now endless process of educational development which is essential for the survival of any profession.'[9]

RESEARCH

'Are we fully equipped in knowledge when we make claims for the therapeutic use of our practice? . . . I would seriously suggest that . . . we concentrate our efforts on some quiet, earnest research work. I think that occupational therapy would stand a very much better chance of attaining recognition as a scientific factor in mental hygiene if we would spend time checking our data and arriving at clear cut decisions as to what were actual facts indicated by inductive methods of search, and what were merely working hypotheses.'[3] This comment was made by Norman Burnette in a paper read in absentia in Atlantic City in 1922, but despite the fact that there was already an awareness of its importance, research did not figure largely in occupational therapy in the early days. Cairns Aitken[1] blames this on the fact that medical rehabilitation frequently arose in response to need; if the response to that need was effective and the practice subsequently became widespread, the moment when scientific evaluation might have been undertaken had passed.

Today there is an increasing awareness among occupational therapists of the need for research. In an article in the *British Journal of Occupational Therapy* entitled 'Why bother to research?'[8] Margaret Ellis, the present chair of the British Association of Occupational Therapists and a former chair of the Research and Degree

Committee of the College of Occupational Therapists, points out that there will never be enough occupational therapists to undertake all the work demanded of them, and that it is therefore important to be certain that the work they do is relevant and based on sound methods.

Claudia Allen [331] emphasizes that theory, practice and research are highly interdependent: an occupational therapist in training learns theory in preparation for clinical practice; once in practice he or she encounters situations that run contrary to theoretical expectation. This 'clinical confusion' can be studied objectively by doing research that in turn may suggest refinements in theory that can then be implemented in practice. She maintains that the process is 'dynamic and circular: from theory to practice to research etc. The absence of any one of these perspectives usually produces an unsatisfactory result, while the presence of all three is exhilarating.'[2] This interdependence is also emphasized by Irwin Lieb and other participants in the papers presented to the national American colloquium, *Occupational therapy education: target 2000*, in 1986 [332].

Under Mrs Ellis's chairmanship of the Research and Degree Committee in the late 1970s, research among occupational therapists was given fresh impetus when negotiations between the committee and the Department of Health and Social Security resulted in the funding of research methods study courses throughout the UK, and in research training fellowships being awarded to members of the remedial professions to help the holders to gain an understanding of the basic principles of research methodology. Details of these fellowships are always announced in the *British Journal of Occupational Therapy*.

The committee also supported research study days, initiated several research editions of the journal and set up an annual research register. This is published in the journal and contains information about ongoing research that has been notified to the College of Occupational Therapists. The College also holds a register of experts in the medical and paramedical fields who have indicated that they would be prepared to advise occupational therapists on research projects. The information is held in a computer database at the college's headquarters and researchers can contact the college to obtain a print-out of others working in their subject or in their geographical area.

The Research Committee exists to help occupational therapists by giving advice on research. Its *Research advice handbook* [348] gives a good basic introduction to research methodology and contains a great deal of practical information: theses available on loan, degree courses open to occupational therapists, relevant Open University courses, societies of interest to occupational therapy researchers and a useful bibliography of books and journals.

Two useful books for occupational therapists and physiotherapists who wish to embark on research or merely to extend their knowledge of the sources available in their field are Smith's *Sources of information on remedial health* [1] and Williams's *Information searching in health care: a workbook for occupational therapists and physiotherapists* [330]. These books and the *Occupational therapists' reference book* [347] provide excellent starting points for anyone interested in finding out more about occupational therapy. As well as being packed with practical information and advice, they will open up a wide field of further sources.

Research methodology for beginners is covered by Partridge and Barnitt [184] and by Bell [338]. Partridge and Barnitt's *Research guidelines* is aimed at practising clinicians who wish to undertake research but lack the appropriate skills. It is a practical and concise guide. Bell covers the whole process of research from planning to report writing with brief checklists of aims and objectives at the end of each chapter. The sections on conducting a literature search and on the principles of questionnaire design are particularly useful. This is a very practical book, well written and presented. Ottenbacher [393] and Payton [553] are for the more advanced researcher and for those who are also interested in the theory and development of research, in the underlying principles and in the different research methods available.

A pattern of training and education in research has now been established in occupational therapy so that research is now regarded as an integral part in the life of an occupational therapist. The special interest groups affiliated to the College of Occupational Therapists and societies such as the Society for Research in Rehabilitation provide opportunities for meeting others involved in research in rehabilitation so that ideas and experiences can be exchanged. 'There is no doubt at all', as the *Research advice handbook* states, 'that the future development of occupational therapy in Great Britain depends on the ability to question, experiment, record, evaluate and, most important of all, communicate its effectiveness.'[5] The special-interest groups affiliated to the college are listed in Part III [1056].

LIBRARIES

Training schools in the UK vary from those within the National Health Service to departments in colleges of further education and polytechnics, and the libraries reflect these differences. Some are specifically oriented towards occupational therapy, with a wide range of relevant material, and cater mainly for occupational therapy students, staff and professionals; others have subject specialist librarians within larger polytechnic, university or medical libraries.

Just as the occupational therapist does not work in isolation, but is part of the paramedical team, so the occupational therapy librarian must be aware of the resources of the wider medical field. There are, however, specific needs and problems relating to the provision of occupational therapy library services, and it was for this reason that the then librarian of the Derby School of Occupational Therapy and the librarian of Dorset House set up the Librarians in Occupational Therapy Schools (LOTS) group in 1984. It was conceived as a support group, a forum for communication between librarians with particular needs and problems. The group meets annually to discuss topics of mutual interest, and a report of their meetings is always published in the *British Journal of Occupational Therapy* [311]. Enquiries should be directed to the chair of the group, at present Sally Croft of the

Dorset House School of Occupational Therapy.

There is no internationally recognized classification scheme specifically for occupational therapy, and the schemes used depend largely on the type of library: university and polytechnic libraries may use Dewey; medical and nursing libraries may use one of the schemes designed for medical libraries, such as the Barnard classification or the National Library of Medicine scheme. Details of these are given in Smith's *Sources of information on remedial health* [1]. Some smaller libraries use their own in-house classification scheme.

GLOSSARIES

Useful glossaries of occupational therapy terminology can be found in a number of books, notably *The occupational therapy manager* [335] pp. 409–10, *Willard and Spackman's Occupational therapy* [369] pp. 836–50, *A model of human occupation* [380] pp. 501–9, *Three frames of reference for mental health* [388] pp. 231–8, *Evaluating clinical change: strategies for occupational and physical therapists* [393] pp. 217–26, and *Therapy as learning* [407] pp. 127–34.

BOOKS

General

There is now a substantial body of literature relating to the principles and practice of occupational therapy. *Willard and Spackman's Occupational therapy* [369], now in its seventh edition and edited by Hopkins and Smith, is a standard reference work. Although it is a textbook written primarily for occupational therapy students, its comprehensive, up-to-date coverage of occupational therapy practice and the underlying theoretical principles make it an invaluable reference tool for all occupational therapists.

Occupational Therapy in the Community

The occupational therapist's role in the community has always been important and is expanding. Bumphrey's book [343] is an excellent introduction to this field. It is a practical book, full of pertinent information, and essential reading for students, practising occupational therapists and, indeed, all those who work in health and welfare. Another useful book is the College of Occupational Therapists' *Resource book for community occupational therapists* [346].

Occupational Therapy for Physical Conditions

Pedretti [396] aims to prepare the student for practice in occupational therapy for adults with acquired physical dysfunction. It is clearly written and well researched

and documented. Trombly [411] presents a compilation of evaluation and therapeutic procedures used in the practice of occupational therapy with physically
disabled adults. Turner [412] is a popular text in British occupational therapy
schools for occupational therapy related to physical disorders.

Occupational Therapy for Psychiatric Conditions

Occupational therapy related to psychiatric conditions is well covered by Willson's
Occupational therapy in long-term psychiatry [416] and her *Occupational therapy in short-
term psychiatry* [417]. These are excellent books, concisely and clearly presented,
invaluable for both students and practising occupational therapists. Hume and
Pullen [371] provide basic information on rehabilitation in psychiatry in a lively
and stimulating form.

The general aim of Finlay's [357] book is to describe the basic theory and
practice of occupational therapy in psychiatry. Her approach shows occupational
therapy as a problem-solving process. Treatment is applied to a wide range of
patients and psychiatric settings, and a case-study form of presentation is used to
illustrate specific treatments and practical application. This book is aimed at both
students and practising occupational therapists and is intended to offer one of the
first comprehensive but practical accounts of the subject.

Allen [331] provides a comprehensive discussion of occupational therapy in
psychiatric practice. The book's purpose, as defined in its preface, is to provide
clear descriptions of mental disorders and of the nature and relative severity of the
cognitive disabilities that accompany these disorders. The book is divided into
three main sections: theory, practice and research.

Denton [354] is a practical text, aimed at students but also applicable to
practising occupational therapists. It outlines current occupational therapy
theories and their specific relationship to practice in mental health settings.

The volume edited by Scott and Katz [408] emphasizes the practical problems
as opposed to the theoretical frameworks. This book is essentially a collection of
occupational therapy experiences from authors who are occupational therapists
from all over the world. Wing and Morris [418] also concentrate on practical
rather than theoretical issues. Their *Handbook of psychiatric rehabilitation practice* is a
manual for all those who staff rehabilitation units for people with chronic
psychiatric disorders.

Remocker and Storch [402] is a manual of exercises for use with small groups of
psychiatric patients, to help them overcome difficulties in effective verbal
communication. It is intended primarily for occupational therapists but will also
prove useful to all those who work with emotionally disturbed patients.

Theoretical Base of Occupational Therapy

In 1970, Anne Cronin Mosey's *Three frames of reference for mental health* [388] was
published. Mosey felt that occupational therapy in psychiatry was functioning on

intuition without a theoretical base. In the preface she puts forward a case for 'the conscious use of theoretical forms of reference as the basis for the treatment of psychosocial dysfunction'. Her book is aimed at students as well as occupational therapists who should be 'continually engaged in rethinking their ideas'.[16] The same author's *Activities therapy* [389] is about the use of work-oriented, recreational and creative-expressive activities as a means of enhancing psychosocial functioning. It focuses on the treatment of adult psychiatric patients and is addressed to both students and practising occupational therapists.

Occupational therapy: configuration of a profession [390] presents a holistic overview of the profession of occupational therapy within the concept of patient management. It helps to clarify how the occupational therapy process contributes to enhancing the functioning of individual patients, and as such is a useful book, not only for students and occupational therapists, but also for those health professionals who collaborate with the occupational therapist. Mosey's concept of a frame of reference as outlined in [388] above is further expanded in her *Psychosocial components of occupational therapy* [391], in which she provides an overview of psychosocial components related to five major areas of specialization in occupational therapy: mental health, physical disabilities, developmental disabilities, gerontology and sensory integration.

Barris *et al.* [336], [337], Briggs and Agrin [341], Bruce and Borg [342] and Hemphill [365] all explore the major theoretical principles on which psychosocial occupational therapy is based and give the contributions and limitations of each frame of reference. They are aimed at practising occupational therapists and at advanced students.

There has been much debate recently within the profession regarding occupational therapy's philosophical base, theoretical concepts and models of practice, and the need to validate practice through well-designed research studies. Kielhofner's *Model of human occupation* [380] makes an important contribution to the development of the concepts and models described by Reilly[18, 19] and Reed [400]. Kielhofner's *Health through occupation* is a stimulating and thought-provoking collection of scholarly arguments, and a very creative, readable and enjoyable book [379]. Howe and Schwartzberg [370] present a new model, specifically for occupational therapy practice, which uses the guide for model development put forward by Reed [400]. This is the functional model, which incorporates the principles of group dynamics and the group theoretical principles of Mosey in her *Activities therapy* [389].

Psychology

Fransella's book [358] is one of a series, the main aims of which are to illustrate how psychology can be applied in particular professional contexts, how it can improve the skills of practitioners and how it can increase both practitioners' and students' understanding of themselves. The majority of the chapters focus on personal and interpersonal psychology. There is a useful chapter on pain, a subject that is also covered by Cromwell [350], whose broad range of articles provides a better understanding of pain, its causes and effects and the ways in which occupational therapists are addressing pain and how to relieve it or live with it.

Counselling

Priestley and McGuire [398] and Priestley *et al.* [399] are both aimed at those who wish to develop their helping skills. Priestley and McGuire covers such skills as interviewing, counselling, information giving and group leading, and would be of use to tutors, training course members and practising workers. Priestley *et al.* is a practical handbook of methods for working with people and helping them to solve their problems. Burnard [344] also offers a practical approach to developing a wide range of counselling skills based on sound theoretical principles. While of great relevance to occupational therapists working with all kinds of disability, these books obviously also have a much more general application.

Creative Therapies

Creative therapies are frequently used with mentally ill patients to encourage self-expression and self-awareness. Warren [413] opens with a discussion of issues general to the creative therapies and then goes on to examine specific activities: the visual arts, dance, music and drama. Relevant games and exercises are included. Jennings [375] explores the therapeutic value of drama with a stimulating collection of ideas that will be of great help to those working with the physically or mentally handicapped and mentally ill, whether children or adults. Liebmann [384] is a useful basic resource for occupational therapists using art in group work, and Landgarten [382] is a good reference source for art therapists, with clear case-studies, a substantial list of references and a bibliography of more than 300 entries.

Physical Rehabilitation

General works on the rehabilitation of physically disabled adults include DeLisa [353], Goodgold [360], O'Sullivan and Schmitz [392], Goodwill and Chamberlain [361] and Granger *et al.* [362]. Goodwill and Chamberlain is intended as a definitive handbook on the rehabilitation of the physically disabled adult, with over 50 chapters covering the major disabling conditions. Written by an interdisciplinary team, it is an important text and reference book for all professional groups concerned with the welfare of handicapped people. DeLisa is aimed at the broad range of health professionals who work with physically disabled people. It covers both basic principles and practical techniques of patient management. Granger *et al.* is written from the point of view of disablement and is designed to introduce students and medical practitioners to the functional approach to medical care.

Rheumatology

In the field of rheumatology, care for the patient with joint disease is at its most effective when there is input from several different professional groups interacting as a team. Melvin [386] concentrates on this team approach. Berry *et al.* [339] emphasizes rehabilitation work as a vital part of the treatment process and stresses the multidisciplinary approach. This book is of value to students as well as to members of the paramedical team. Clarke [345] is also aimed at members of the rehabilitation team. It covers all aspects of care from clinical indications and drug treatments to the roles of each team member in the long-term rehabilitation of patients at home and in the community.

Hand and Upper Limb

Mills and Fraser [387] concentrate on the rehabilitation of people with injuries of the upper limb. This is a practical manual with each therapeutic activity accompanied by a task analysis and an illustration. Salter [404] is practice-orientated, covering many aspects of hand rehabilitation. It is well laid out with good photographs and is useful for all therapists involved in the rehabilitation of people with hand injuries, as well as for students.

Paediatrics

The role of the occupational therapist in paediatrics has developed considerably during the 1980s. In part this is because of changing attitudes to disabled people and a growing awareness of the physical, psychological and social needs of both the disabled child and the child's family. Penso [397] is both a guide for the practising occupational therapist and a textbook for the student. It concentrates on how to help children with disabilities cope with necessary daily living skills, and stresses the importance of the child's environment and the need for advising and counselling parents. Axline [334] demonstrates the value of play therapy with children who are emotionally disturbed. The book, with its case-histories, will interest parents, occupational therapists and anyone concerned with the growth and development of children. McCarthy [385] is full of information and practical advice for all professionals who are in contact with the physically handicapped child, and Knickerbocker [381] is an excellent and practical book for use by a wide range of people who are involved with children with learning disabilities.

Mental Handicap

Occupational therapy, with its client-centred approach, has an important role to play in helping mentally handicapped people to live a full and satisfying life within the community. Hogg and Raynes [366] covers the important area of assessment in mental handicap and the variety of techniques involved. Shanley [409] is directed towards those who have day-to-day contact with mentally handicapped people and towards students preparing to work with them. The emphasis throughout is on the practical means of improving quality of life. Similarly, Peck and Chia [395] concentrates less on explaining mental handicap and more on developing an integrated approach to the teaching of independent living skills. Services for mentally handicapped people are changing in favour of care within the community and this area of involvement for occupational therapists is covered by Isaac [372].

The Elderly

The large and growing ageing population forms a fundamental part of the profession of occupational therapy. Helm [364] is a well-presented, comprehensive and informative book that would be useful for any occupational therapist involved with the care of the elderly. Crepeau [349] emphasizes that old age should be a stimulating period of growth and development and not one of apathy and dependence. This comprehensive book will help occupational therapists to design an activity programme to meet the needs of elderly people in their care. Squires's *Rehabilitation of the older patient* [410] is one of Croom Helm's Therapy in Practice series (now published by Chapman & Hall). Squires adopts a positive attitude to the rehabilitation of the older person and emphasizes the team approach. Holden and Woods's *Reality orientation* [368], a well-established text, is a practical working manual, which clearly describes the principles and techniques of this widely used method of treating confusion, disorientation and memory loss in the elderly. Jacques [373] is aimed at all those who care for or are involved with dementia sufferers. This does not set out to be a practical manual but is intended to be a guide to understanding the problems of dementia. Holden's *Thinking it through* [367] is a short, thought-provoking handbook that reviews key points for enhancing the physical and psychological environment of the elderly. It is published by the Winslow Press [1312], which has a wide selection of books, resource packs, photographs and slides relating to the care of the elderly. A very detailed catalogue is available from the Winslow Press.

Neurology

The field of neurology is a stimulating one and can present occupational therapists with a wide variety of diseases and disorders affecting the nervous systems. Occupational therapy's holistic approach – the ability to see not just the disorder, but the person involved, with all his or her physical, functional, psychological and social needs – is especially appropriate. Eggers [355] considers in detail the sensorimotor disability of hemiplegic patients and its treatment in occupational therapy. Although particular attention is devoted to the upper limb in the activities of daily living, the rehabilitation of the whole person is always kept in sight. This is a practical book, based on the Bobath principle. Fussey and Giles [359] stresses a practical, interdisciplinary approach to the rehabilitation of the severely brain-injured adult. The emphasis is on the basic aim of the development of functional skills for independent living. Wilcock [415] provides an invaluable discussion of the principles and techniques of the different approaches to stroke and gives a practical basis for treatment for occupational therapists both in training and in practice.

Johnstone [377], [378] provides a clear, straightforward practical approach to the rehabilitation of the stroke patient. Johnstone is a physiotherapist, but she stresses that successful rehabilitation is very much a team effort, and there is much in both books that would be relevant to occupational therapists. Her *Home care of the stroke patient* [376] concentrates on helping the patient and family to understand their role in the recovery of the patient. All three books are well and clearly illustrated. Schwartz [407] is a book that is relevant to those working with patients with neurological impairments. Schwartz integrates theoretical concepts and therapeutic application and presents his findings in a clear and interesting manner.

Management

All occupational therapists are faced with the challenge of providing the best possible service given the resources available at their command. De Gilio *et al.* [340] is a key text that is designed to help occupational therapists meet the new management challenges and acquire and develop new skills. It is essentially a practical manual, and its convenient ringbound form and large A4 format make it ideal for use in training sessions and workshops. Bair and Gray [335] provides a comprehensive introduction to management in occupational therapy. It is aimed at new, inexperienced managers, as well as providing guidelines for established practitioners in management positions. Andamo [333] contains selected readings on programme evaluation and quality assurance and is aimed at administrators. Ellis [356] is aimed at professionals, managers, teachers and academics. While not an easy book to read, it is stimulating and well worth the effort for anyone with a serious interest in quality assurance.

CURRENT AWARENESS SOURCES, INDEXES AND ABSTRACTS

Since occupational therapists are involved in a wide variety of fields, many of the well-known indexes to medical literature and the principal guides and abstracting services will prove useful sources of information. Barbara Smith's *Sources of information on remedial health* [1] is particularly helpful in detailing these. There is, however, comparatively little of this kind of information specifically for occupational therapy. As a result of requests from the profession, the Medical Information Service of the British Library decided to add occupational therapy to its series of current awareness topics searches (CATS) [78]. These are keyword and author indexed lists of current journal references taken from over 100 key journals and dating back to late 1986. The lists appear monthly and are generally much more up to date than many 'current awareness' listings; they contain much bibliographic material not covered by other medical indexing services. Two other indexes issued more recently by the Medical Information Service are also particularly relevant for occupational therapists: *Rehabilitation Index* [80] covers disability, handicap, physical diseases and injuries, mental disorders, rehabilitation methods and equipment, rehabilitation education and service management; *Terminal Care Index* [81] covers care of the terminally ill, hospices, palliative treatment, treatment of intractable pain, attitudes to death and dying and coping with bereavement. Many of the other titles produced by the Medical Information Service are also relevant, for example, those on dementia, alcoholism, depression, schizophrenia, psychiatry in old age and psychotherapy.

The National Centre for Training and Education in Prosthetics and Orthotics at the University of Strathclyde maintains a library and information service. It publishes a fortnightly current awareness list, *RECAL (Rehabilitation Engineering Current Awareness List)* [228], which lists articles from over 100 journals taken by the centre, copies of which may be obtained directly from them. Among the subjects covered are prosthetics, orthotics, wheelchairs, seating for the disabled, aids for the physically disabled and biomechanics. Their *RECAL Abstracts* service offers a bi-annual compilation of additions to the *RECAL* database and all articles include a factual abstract and indexing terms. A new service, *RECAL Offline* [422], offers the centre's database of more than 14 000 bibliographic records to the subscriber for use in his or her own place of work. The centre also undertakes literature searches on request and makes these available to subscribers.

The *Rehabilitation Bulletin* [92], produced monthly by the National Demonstration Centre at the Department of Neurology and Neurosurgery and Neurological Trauma at Pinderfields General Hospital, is another useful source of recent journal citations on the rehabilitation of physical handicap. It also lists new books and audiovisual publications received by the centre and gives notice of forthcoming events.

The British Institute of Mental Handicap whose concern is the improvement of care for mentally handicapped people both in hospital and in the community, has an information and resource centre to answer queries on all aspects of mental handicap. It also operates a monthly Current Awareness Service [324] to keep those who are interested abreast of the latest books and articles relating to mental handicap. The service covers over 300 sources from the UK, the rest of Europe, North America, Australia and New Zealand. The Disabled Living Foundation and Disability Scotland do not produce lists of journal articles, but their regularly updated information lists [156], [325] offer a current awareness service on aids currently available, recently published books, and associations that exist to help disabled people.

The Library Association has recently introduced a new service with its *Applied Social Sciences Index and Abstracts (ASSIA)* [86]. It is international in scope with over

500 journals from 16 countries and covers the whole range of the 'caring services'. *ASSIA* comes out six times a year and cumulates into one annual sequence. The method of organization is very straightforward and the quality of the abstracts is high.

JOURNALS

The *Occupational Therapy Index* [78] mentioned above indexes over 100 key journals; only a few of these are mentioned here. The *British Journal of Occupational Therapy* [311] is the official journal of the College of Occupational Therapists and appears monthly. In addition to articles of a clinical nature on a wide variety of subjects, including research, it contains many items of general interest to its readers, with job vacancies, letters, book reviews, news about the World Federation of Occupational Therapists and a calendar of coming events that gives details of courses, study days and regional meetings. The official journals of the American, Australian and Canadian associations, the *American Journal of Occupational Therapy* [308], the *Australian Occupational Therapy Journal* [310] and the *Canadian Journal of Occupational Therapy* [312], have a format similar to that of the British journal.

Therapy Weekly [53], the UK's only weekly newspaper for the remedial professions, is distributed to physiotherapists, occupational therapists and speech therapists at their places of work. It contains the latest information on matters affecting the professions as well as job vacancies and book reviews.

Some journals that concentrate on specific areas of interest to occupational therapists are *Design for Special Needs, Radar Bulletin, Contact, PIP Newsletter, OTSIGN Newsletter* and *OT Micronews. Design for Special Needs* [314] is published by the Centre on Environment for the Handicapped. The centre's main area of concern is housing design and access and this is reflected in its monthly journal. *Radar Bulletin* [323] and *Contact* [313] are both published by RADAR (the Royal Association for Disability and Rehabilitation), *Contact* monthly in magazine format and *Radar Bulletin* 11 times per year in the form of a newsletter. The *Bulletin* gives up-to-date information of interest to disabled people on government legislation, employment, education, housing, mobility, aids and equipment, and events and conferences. *Contact* covers similar topics, but is in a magazine format with articles rather than news.

PIP Newsletter [322] is the newsletter of the Paediatric Interest People, a special-interest group affiliated to the College of Occupational Therapists. Although the group is open to all professions working in the field of paediatrics, the majority of the members are occupational therapists and the group considers itself predominantly an occupational therapy group. Their newsletter is issued three times per year and contains letters, notices of coming events and book reviews, as well as stimulating and varied articles on different aspects of paediatrics. Another special-interest group that has grown into a national group is OTSIGN (Occupational

Therapy Special Interest Group in Neurology). Its main aim is to provide support and continuing education in occupational therapy for neurological conditions. The newsletter [319] is published twice a year and gives details of book reviews, relevant associations, courses and workshops as well as case-studies.

Details of all special interest groups affiliated to the College of Occupational Therapists are given in Part III [1056]. Many of them produce newsletters and all will respond to direct enquiry.

American journals include the *Occupational Therapy Journal of Research* [317], which was first published in 1981 by the American Occupational Therapy Foundation and reflects the awareness of the growing importance of research, and the Haworth Press's *Occupational Therapy in Health Care* [315]. This was launched in 1984 as a thematic quarterly journal. Under the editorship of Florence Cromwell each issue concentrates on one broad topic with articles by practising occupational therapists. The Haworth Press also publishes *Occupational Therapy in Mental Health* [316], *Physical and Occupational Therapy in Pediatrics* [321] and *Physical and Occupational Therapy in Geriatrics* [320].

The previous decade had seen the publication of two international scientific journals devoted to disability and handicap. These were *International Rehabilitation Medicine*, now called *International Disability Studies*, and the *International Journal of Rehabilitation Research*. *International Disability Studies* [44] is issued quarterly. It describes itself as encouraging 'work on all aspects of disablement, with the aim of promoting greater and more sensitive appreciation of and response to the reality of disability, primarily by publication of original research-based papers'. It contains a calendar of meetings and events world-wide. The *International Journal of Rehabilitation Research* [45] is published quarterly, with original contributions in English, German or French, and with summaries in English, German, French and Spanish. Other information is given in English. This is the journal in which abstracts of the Society for Research in Rehabilitation have been regularly published. These abstracts are now published in *Clinical Rehabilitation* [41], a more recent (1987) international journal that emphasizes the dissemination of practical approaches to rehabilitation, the exchange of ideas and the presentation of research relevant to clinical practice. These three journals are excellent sources of up-to-date information on research papers and projects.

AIDS AND EQUIPMENT

Equally important for the occupational therapist is literature relating to the various aids and equipment available for disabled people. Disability Scotland and the Disabled Living Foundation in England and Wales offer similar comprehensive services for all those concerned with disabled people, whether they are professionals, voluntary organizations or individuals requiring up-to-date information about aids, equipment and services. The organizations have extensive information banks on all aspects of disability except for the purely medical, and, as well as responding to direct enquiry, they publish regularly updated information lists [155], [325] that contain details of aids, equipment, facilities and services for disabled people. In Northern Ireland the Disabled Living Foundation's information lists are distributed by the Northern Ireland Information Service for Disabled People.

Disability Scotland has linked up with the Disabled Living Foundation's aids and equipment database and has extended it to include information on holidays and voluntary organizations and Scottish suppliers. It makes this information accessible to subscribers using basic desktop or portable computers [423]. This facility has been created to provide a better service for people with disabilities by making it available to social work departments and health boards, who can call up the central computer and receive immediate up-to-date information on these subjects.

The information in the lists put out by Disability Scotland and the Disabled Living Foundation is obtained from the manufacturers and is not therefore independently evaluated. The *Equipment for the disabled* series [157], however, does supply independent and professional information about the wide range of aids and equipment available today. These fully illustrated, authoritative guides also offer advice on selection and suggest solutions to various problems which might arise. Most of the equipment shown has been used by a disabled person and its use assessed by a therapist.

The Department of Health sponsors and finances a programme to provide for the assessment of equipment in use by disabled people in a practical way, as distinct from evaluation under normal research conditions. The findings of this Disability Equipment Assessment Programme [432] (formerly the DHSS Aids Assessment Programme) are published regularly and supplied free of charge to those who are interested.

There are several books of information on aids available that while of use to professionals, are mainly aimed at disabled people and their carers. Darnbrough and Kinrade's *Directory of aids for disabled and elderly people* [352] aims to make basic information directly available to disabled people themselves. As is the case with these authors' *Directory for disabled people* [153], all information is derived from source. Weyers [414] concentrates on providing information specifically on wheelchairs. *With a little help* [363] was written by the Muscular Dystrophy Group's occupational therapist and intended primarily to include aids that are relevant to the problems of muscular dystrophy and allied neuromuscular diseases, but the book is useful for people with a wider range of disabilities. Jay [374] is a comprehensive and easy-to-read guide on ways of overcoming the difficulties of disabilities in everyday life. Although these books are written for disabled people, the authors all stress the importance of obtaining professional advice and of working closely with an occupational therapist or with a trained adviser at a Disabled Living Centre to avoid wasted time, effort and money.

In 1983 the Scottish Home and Health Department set up a Committee for Research on Equipment for the Disabled (CRED) to advise the chief scientist of the SHHD on research, development and evaluation of technical aids for loco-motor and physical disability. One of its functions was to determine those areas where improvements could be made to existing aids and where there was a need for the development of new aids. In 1988 it published its report, *A survey of aids and equipment for disabled people in Scotland* [458].

The Handicapped Persons Research Unit at the Newcastle upon Tyne Poly-technic publishes papers on information on special needs. As a result of the success of these papers the unit has set up the British database on research into aids for the disabled (*BARD*) [420]. The main aim is to improve and facilitate the exchange of ideas and information at the research and design stage of production of aids and equipment. The database, which has been operational since 1984, contains over 1000 records on British design and development works, prototypes, one-offs, details of research projects, surveys and evaluations. Information is supplied through print-outs in response to specific enquiries and through reports on partic-ular descriptions of aids. The unit also produces *The concerned technology* [405], a directory that gives details of the wide variety of electronic aids now available to help people of all ages who have special needs. It contains a useful bibliography of further reading.

MICROCOMPUTERS

A more recent development is the *BARDSOFT* database [421], which is entirely devoted to software for special needs and contains information on over 1000 programs for over 40 types of microcomputer. This is a fast-growing area of treat-ment in occupational therapy. In 1983 the Department of Health and Social Security and the Department of Trade and Industry inaugurated a scheme to place BBC microcomputers in hospital occupational therapy departments and social service department day centres in the UK. The equipment and software were provided by the Department of Trade and Industry's Information Technology Awareness Programme, and the intention was to use the computers as therapeutic and assessment aids. It was thought that some areas in particular might lend themselves to treatment by computer: the restoration of digital and upper limb function following trauma; the retraining of brain-damaged patients; motivational and recreational use by long-stay accident victims, and the possibil-ity of work training or some vocational retraining were identified as possible areas in which a computer might prove valuable.

In order to support occupational therapy microcomputer users the College of Occupational Therapists and the DHSS co-operated in initiating a newsletter, *OT Micronews* [318]. The newsletter is an invaluable source of information on current projects and the use of microcomputers in occupational therapy, and includes use-ful book reviews and reading lists. It is available by subscription only. A national Special Interest Group in Microcomputers was set up 'to share and disseminate information on computer technology as applied in occupational therapy'.[7]

It is obviously important that students in occupational therapy schools and, indeed, practising occupational therapists who qualified before microcomputers were in general use, should be familiar with microcomputers and their therapeutic use so that they are well aware of the range of possible applications and are able to exploit its potential to the full when working with patients. There has been a recent increase in literature on the use of the microcomputer in occupational therapy and on microcomputer-based aids for the disabled.

In 1986 Shena Latto, a Senior Research Fellow at the College of Occupational Therapy in Liverpool, produced a report on the use of microcomputers in occupational therapy [383]. The proposal for this descriptive study had been submitted to the DHSS in 1981 at the commencement of the DHSS/DTI scheme. It describes the DHSS/DTI initiative and records the information generated by the exercise. It gives information about computer use in occupational therapy departments throughout the country, information about particular departments in psychiatry, physical handicap and mental handicap, and also presents individual case histories that give a picture of treatment applications for occupational therapists planning departmental programmes.

Another book aimed at practising occupational therapists is Cromwell's *Computer applications in occupational therapy* [351], although its relevance is more for the occupational therapist who already has some computer experience. The papers that deal with specific applications of the microcomputer are particularly useful. Both Saunders [406] and Ridgway and McKears [403] will be of interest to disabled people themselves, as well as to occupational therapists who have little or no experience of microcomputers.

The information lists produced by Disability Scotland [325] and the Disabled Living Foundation [156] give further titles, as does the *Occupational therapists' reference book* [347], and it is worth contacting the appropriate special-interest group [1056], which will be aware of computer applications relevant to its field of interest. There are now few fields in which the computer cannot play a useful part in the rehabilitation of the patient.

VOLUNTARY ORGANIZATIONS AND STATUTORY BODIES

Besides keeping up to date with current literature and journal articles, with aids and equipment, with computer projects and software, the occupational therapist must have a knowledge of social and economic problems as they affect the patient, and of work opportunities. It is therefore necessary to keep abreast of the benefits and services available for disabled people and to be aware of the groups, societies and statutory and voluntary organizations that exist to help them.

In the UK the Department of Health and Social Security and the Scottish Home and Health Department both publish leaflets with information of special interest to disabled people – a list can be found in the *Occupational therapists' reference book* [347]. Information about government policy as it affects disabled people can be found in *Radar Bulletin* [323], published by the Royal Association for Disability and Rehabilitation. RADAR is the United Kingdom representative of Rehabilitation International and acts as a co-ordinating body for the voluntary groups serving disabled people. It is able to supply information on a wide range of subjects, including housing, holidays and government legislation. It is particularly active in promoting better access to public buildings and has published a number of access guides. Its invaluable publications list contains a number of books, pamphlets and other literature relating to the whole range of disability information.

The Centre on Environment for the Handicapped [1129] provides a specialist information and advisory service on the environmental needs of all handicapped people. It is concerned not just with the physical environment, with housing and access, but also with discrimination shown to disabled people by individual attitudes and by local and national government policies.

The Disability Alliance [1131] is a federation of organizations of and for people with disabilities who have joined together to press for a comprehensive income scheme for disabled people. It offers information and advice on matters relating to finance and benefits and the financial implications of disability. Its *Disability rights handbook* [164], published annually, is subtitled 'a guide to rights, benefits and services for all people with disabilities and their families'. Darnbrough and Kinrade refer to it as 'a much used and much respected guide specifically for people with disabilities. It has the merit of being relatively inexpensive while being sufficiently detailed to cope with most day to day problems.'[6]

Voluntary organizations are playing an increasingly important role both in providing help, advice and support to those who use them and in facilitating communication between the patient and the professional. There is much more emphasis now on 'care within the community' and the voluntary organizations complement and extend the services provided by the statutory agencies.

There are several books on the market that give lists of voluntary organizations and self-help groups, but since contact addresses, especially of smaller groups, change frequently, they are often already out of date. Disability Scotland issues regularly updated lists [325] of voluntary organizations as part of its information service, and the Disabled Living Foundation publishes information papers [156] on organizations and information sources for disabled people. Darnbrough and Kinrade's *Directory for disabled people* [153] is also a useful source. This is a most thorough and authoritative handbook of information and opportunities for disabled and handicapped people. It is continually revised and the authors say in their introduction that they try 'to cover every new development, leaving no stone unturned to ensure that nothing which might be of benefit to a disabled person is missed'.[6] This book is an indispensable reference tool for disabled people, their families and the professional.

DIAL UK [1130], the National Association of Disablement Information and Advice services, is a growing organization of local self-help groups, all of which offer a free, impartial and confidential service of information, advice and, in some cases, practical help, provided by people with direct personal experience of disability. It has a network of local DIAL groups and information about them can be obtained from DIAL House in Chesterfield.

The Help for Health scheme, run and funded by the Wessex Regional Health Authority, is a computerized system with a database [424] containing details of over 3000 mainly English self-help organizations, more than 2000 leaflets and pamphlets and at least 800 publications. The Scottish equivalent, Health Search Scotland [425], operated by the Scottish Health Education Group, has been available to the public since May 1989. These services are particularly useful for maintaining up-to-date information on local support groups where contact names, addresses and telephone numbers tend to change more frequently than in the bigger organizations.

With these sources available, this book does not attempt to list all the various organizations that exist to help disabled people. Such a list would be a long one since, as Darnbrough and Kinrade say, 'It must be true to say that there are few problems for which a society has not been established to try to solve the difficulty.'[6]

References

1. Aitken, C. (1988). Research and development in rehabilitation. In Gooodwill, C. J. and Chamberlain, M. A. (eds), *Rehabilitation of the physically disabled adult*. London: Croom Helm.
2. Allen, C. (1985). *Occupational therapy for psychiatric diseases*. Boston: Little, Brown & Co.
3. Burnette, N. (1923). The status of occupational therapy in Canada. *Archives of Occupational Therapy*, **2** (3), 179–83.
4. Commemorative issue (1986). *Canadian Journal of Occupational Therapy*, **53** (November).
5. College of Occupational Therapists. (1985). *Research advice handbook*. London: COT.
6. Darnbrough, A. and Kinrade, D. (1985). *Directory for disabled people*, 4th edn. London: Woodhead-Faulkner.
7. Editorial (1984). *OT Micronews*, **1** (1), 1.
8. Ellis, M. (1981). Why bother to research? *British Journal of Occupational Therapy*, **44** (4), 115–16.
9. Green, M. (1988). Planning for change in education. *British Journal of Occupational Therapy*, **51** (3), 78–80.
10. Groundes-Peace, Z. (1957). An outline of the development of occupational therapy in Scotland. *Scottish Journal of Occupational Therapy*, **30**, 1–22.
11. *Hansard*, 28 July 1989, 1428, 1429.
12. Hopkins, H. L. (1988). An historical perspective in occupational therapy. In Hopkins, H. L. and Smith, H. D (eds), *Willard and Spackman's Occupational therapy*, 7th edn. Philadelphia: J. B. Lippincott.
13. Licht, S. (1948). *Occupational therapy source book*. Baltimore: Williams & Wilkins.

14. Macdonald, E. (1960). The evolution of the techniques used in occupational therapy and the place of the treatment in the social and therapeutic services of today. In Macdonald, E. (ed.), *Occupational therapy in rehabilitation*. London: Baillière, Tindall & Cox.

15. Mendez, A. (1988). *A chronicle of the World Federation of Occupational Therapists. The first thirty years 1952–1982*. World Federation of Occupational Therapists (available from the College of Occupational Therapists, London).

16. Mosey, A. C. (1970). *Three frames of reference for mental health*. Thorofare, NJ: C. B. Slack.

17. Pinel, P. (1801). Medical philosophical treatise on mental alienation. Paris. In Licht, S. (1948). *Occupational therapy source book*. Baltimore: Williams & Wilkins.

18. Reilly, M. (1962). Occupational therapy can be one of the great ideas of twentieth century medicine. *American Journal of Occupational Therapy*, **16**, 1–9.

19. Reilly, M. (1969). The education process. *American Journal of Occupational Therapy*, **23**, 299–307.

6 Physiotherapy

Graham Walton

INTRODUCTION

In the United Kingdom there are over 22 000 chartered physiotherapists working in the private sector and the National Health Service. The only recognized examining and professional body for physiotherapists in the UK is the Chartered Society of Physiotherapy (CSP). At present it has 75 branches spread throughout the UK. At international level 44 national physiotherapy organizations make up the membership of the World Confederation for Physical Therapy. This was formed in 1948 with the objectives of sharing benefits, learning and help and also strengthening international professional links.

HISTORY

Throughout the ages various techniques of physiotherapy have been used in many countries, including ancient China, Egypt and Greece. Massage and gymnastic methods were described 5000 years ago in the Kong Fu Chinese records. Hippocrates wrote in 380 BC, 'A physician must be experienced in many things but assuredly also in rubbing.' The Roman physician Galen recommended massage for certain injuries in AD 200. Hydrotherapy was another therapy that was evident in some form in the days of the Roman Empire. In the nineteenth century the Swede, Henreich Ling, devised a physiologically based system of massage and exercise. Niels Finsen, a Danish physician, discovered the therapeutic value of actinic rays in the same century.

The term 'physiotherapy' was first used on 15 July 1905 in a letter in the *British Medical Journal*. In the UK the profession emerged when the Society of Trained Masseuses was established in 1894. The Royal Charter was granted to an organization called the Chartered Society of Massage and Remedial Gymnasts in 1920. The profession eventually became the Chartered Society of Physiotherapy in 1943. After the Dutch, it is the second oldest physiotherapy professional organization in the world. In the USA the discipline is known as 'physical therapy'. Ramsden[24] has traced the profession's development there and found that the first national meeting took place in 1922.

DEFINITION

Despite this long history a major issue facing physiotherapy is the need for a precise definition of the professional role. This lack of clarity has been addressed by Nunley[20] and Williams.[30] The 1920 Royal Charter describes therapists as 'persons engaged in the practice of massage, medical gymnastics and electrotherapy or kindred methods of treatment'. Williams[30] argues that this definition is still pertinent, with the three components – massage, medical gymnastics and medical electricity – still being central. A discussion article entitled 'The practice of physiotherapy'[23] was published in 1988 to try to promote debate on the definition of physiotherapy. Among the issues discussed as being relevant to physiotherapy were communication and research skills and the need for clinical assessments.

RESEARCH AWARENESS

The importance of research into physiotherapy practice is beginning to be recognized, at least in the literature. Atkinson[4] and Harrison[17] describe the need for a scientific knowledge basis for physiotherapy. In a wide-reaching article Peat[22] suggests that the profession will only survive and progress through increased research programmes. He also underlines the need for physiotherapists to report their work through publishing. A comprehensive description of how to evaluate and appraise research reports has been written by Parry.[21] The American Physical Therapy Association has produced guidelines on how to evaluate research papers.[1] Domholdt and Malone[12] also look at evaluating research and include an annotated bibliography relating to research.

Despite this growing awareness there still appears to be a reluctance to undertake or read physiotherapy research. Some of the reasons for this are outlined in an editorial by Rothstein.[26] Grabois and Fuhrer[16] completed a survey of physiatrists' views on conducting research. There were 550 usable returns (a response rate of 43 per cent), which showed that only 2 per cent were spending more than a quarter of their time on research.

A more positive picture emerges in a citation frequency study of two physio-therapy journals.[11] There was found to be a correlation between physiotherapists considered eminent by practitioners and those with high frequency ratings. The authors concluded that this illustrates the transition to a more scientifically oriented profession from a practice-based profession. An analysis of articles[10] published in *Physiotherapy Canada* [467] found that there was a 12 per cent increase in data based articles and a 20 per cent decrease in descriptive articles between 1977 and 1982, compared with articles published between 1973 and 1976.

INFORMATION USE

Bunch[8] describes two research studies by Lloyd (a physiotherapist) and Fraser (a librarian), and Smith (a librarian) into the information needs of physiotherapists. They reveal that information is required by the physiotherapist for: personal in-service training and continuing education/current awareness; education and training of others at all levels; support for day-to-day work; information to pass on to patients and their families; and information to keep abreast of equipment development and availability.

Dyer[13] describes how using libraries, journals and other relevant literature contributes to professional development. Various chapters have appeared that explain and describe information skills and information sources for the physiotherapist.[9, 28] The need for library and information skills is becoming recognized in the physiotherapy students' curriculum. An information skills workbook for physiotherapy students at McMaster University, Ontario, is described by Williams *et al*.[31]

The need for physiotherapy management information concerning manpower, treatment activity and financial costs has become recognized in the United Kingdom since 1987, with the Körner report [560]. The implications and implementation of this report are discussed in two articles in *Physiotherapy*.[19, 27] Despite this, there is a low level of specialized library and information facilities for the physiotherapist.[2] Library provisions do exist for physiotherapy students in their institutions, whether they be hospital based or studying in higher education. Qualified physiotherapists do not always have access to these resources. Harrison[17] has observed the lack of a research library at the headquarters of the Chartered Society of Physiotherapy. In 1989 this deficiency was remedied with the appointment of a research and liaison officer, who will have responsibility for a research information service.

Specialized library facilities are available in the United Kingdom from some multi-disciplinary hospital libraries. Health authorities that have a regional library network service can also meet the physiotherapists' information needs. One initiative that might point to the future is the setting up of a library network for the sharing of disability and rehabilitation literature in Canada.[18]

PHYSIOTHERAPY LITERATURE

The acceleration of scientific growth and the resulting increase in publications has been well documented. Peat[7] questioned in 1981 whether physiotherapy had kept pace with this growth rate. Before the 1950s, physiotherapy textbooks were written by other professionals. One of the first textbooks to be produced by a physiotherapist and for physiotherapists was Joan Cash's *Physiotherapy in medical conditions* in 1951. Since 1981 there have been significant developments. Some publishers produce series of books specifically on physiotherapy (Churchill Livingstone's 'Clinics in Physical Therapy' and 'International Perspectives in Physical Therapy'). Most physiotherapy textbooks are now written solely by physiotherapists or have some contribution from a physiotherapist. There have also appeared major new physiotherapy periodical titles (*Clinical Management in Physical Therapy* [470] and *Physiotherapy Practice* [471]).

JOURNALS

The range of advantages physiotherapy journals have over other sources of information have been examined by Arnell.[3] They are one of the most accessible sources of current information for the clinician. They can be relied upon for accuracy more than can personal experience and opinion. Most physiotherapy journals were linked with professional bodies but the past decade has seen the commencement of significant new titles.

Before World War I the only two physiotherapy journals were *Physiotherapy* [460] and the *Nederlands Tijdschrift voor Fysiotherapie* [461]: the official journal of the Chartered Society of Physiotherapy in the UK and the Dutch equivalent. In the following years various countries' professional physiotherapy associations started publishing their own journals. These included *American Journal of Physical Medicine and Rehabilitation* [462], *Archives of Physical Medicine and Rehabilitation* [463] (American Congress of Rehabilitation Medicine), *Australian Journal of Physiotherapy* [464], *Physical Therapy* [465] (American Physical Therapy Association), *Physiotherapie* [466] (Germany), *Physiotherapy Canada* [467] and the *South African Journal of Physiotherapy* [468]. A Scandinavian English language journal intended both for the physician and the physiotherapist was also started: the *Scandinavian Journal of Rehabilitation Medicine* [52].

A specialized physiotherapy journal that commenced in the 1970s is the *Journal of Orthopaedic and Sports Physical Therapy* [469]. The aim of *Clinical Management in Physical Therapy* [470] is to concentrate on articles based more on experience and observation than research. The peer-reviewed *Physiotherapy Practice* [471] commenced publication in 1984. *Physical Therapy in Health Care* [472] is a review journal concentrating on a single topic per issue. Reviews and physiotherapy research are covered in the multi-disciplinary *Clinical Rehabilitation* [41].

Two important articles by Bohannon, entitled 'Citation analysis of *Physical*

Therapy'[7] and 'Core journals of physiotherapy',[5] are the results of studies to identify the core physiotherapy journals. In the first article, all reference lists in *Physical Therapy* between June 1980 and May 1984 were analysed to record the citation frequency of various journals. Over 40 per cent of the references cited were from only 15 journals out of the 676 journals cited in total. In the second article, the survey was expanded in 1986 to include four citing physiotherapy journals. Some consistency did emerge but there was a lack of absolute uniformity.

CURRENT AWARENESS SERVICES

One indication of the increase in physiotherapy journal titles is the production of the *Physiotherapy Index* [79] by the Medical Information Service of the British Library Document Supply Centre. Roberts[25] has described the setting up of this publication. It is compiled from 100 journals that often include physiotherapy-related material as well as from 3 000 other biomedical journals. Bohannon[6] has concluded that the *Physiotherapy Index* [79] is 'excellent for keeping up to date'. The non-cumulative nature and lack of annual index are disadvantages for retrospective searching.

The Institute for Scientific Information in the USA produces a series of current awareness publications called *Current Contents*. The three with most relevance to physiotherapy are *Clinical Medicine* [473], *Life Sciences* [474] and *Social and Behavioral Sciences* [475]. The contents pages of a variety of relevant journals and books are reproduced soon after publication. There is an author index and address directory, and a subject index based on the natural language in the article titles in each weekly issue. Stewart[28] has pointed out that as it is 'air-freighted from the USA for rapid distribution in Europe it generally reproduces the contents before the journals themselves get into the country'. Physiotherapy is not among the subject groupings and the only specific physiotherapy journal title included is *Physical Therapy* [465].

Another source of current information is the professional physiotherapy journal. *Physiotherapy* [460] includes a section that lists selected contents from a range of physiotherapy and related journals. There are informative abstracts of relevant articles written for inclusion in *Physical Therapy* [465]. The bibliographical details of recommended journal articles are included in *Physiotherapy Canada* [467].

INDEXES AND ABSTRACTS

Unlike the case of current awareness services, for which there is *Physiotherapy Index* [79], there is no specific indexing or abstracting service on physiotherapy. Over 2700 journal titles are used by the National Library of Medicine to compile *Index Medicus* [58]. Again, *Physical Therapy* [465] is the only strictly physiotherapy journal title represented but many of the other titles are relevant. *Index Medicus* [58] has been issued since 1879 and now comes out monthly with annual cumulations. Bibliographic references are organized using a list of index terms entitled *Medical Subject Headings (MeSH)* [60]. It is essential that when using *Index Medicus* this thesaurus is consulted for the most appropriate heading. 'Physical therapy' is the main specific heading with others of relevance being 'exercise therapy', 'hydrotherapy', 'massage' and 'ultraviolet therapy'. The subject entries in *Index Medicus* [58] are arranged using subheadings that include anatomy, aetiology, methods and occurrence. When looking for management-related material, *Hospital Literature Index* [88] is suitable. Under the main heading physical therapy there are subheadings on such areas as education, manpower and standards.

In comparison to the one physiotherapy journal included in *Index Medicus* [58], the *Cumulative Index to Nursing and Allied Health (CINAHL)* [69] uses at least 10 relevant titles. Another 350 journals are also incorporated in *CINAHL*, which is organized using a thesaurus based on MeSH. The other journals used in compiling *CINAHL* are from nursing and allied health subjects. This results in physiotherapy-related material published in medical journals being omitted.

The major abstracting service for the physiotherapist is published by the Excerpta Medica Foundation [65]. *Excerpta Media* has 46 individual printed sections with one entitled *Rehabilitation and Physical Therapy* [476], which is issued 10 times a year. Over 4000 journals are used including at least six physiotherapy titles. There is an author and subject index in each issue, with abstracts arranged in subject groupings that include anatomy and physiotherapy. A cumulative annual index is also produced.

Two other abstracting publications relevant to the physiotherapist are *Applied Social Sciences Index and Abstracts (ASSIA)* and *Health Service Abstracts*. *ASSIA* [86] is notable for its broad subject coverage of the psychosocial areas, which compensates for the non-inclusion of physiotherapy journal titles. *Health Service Abstracts* [71] is useful for management literature and includes physiotherapy as a subject heading.

REFERENCE BOOKS

There are only a few reference books published specifically for the physiotherapist. One of these is the *Chartered physiotherapists' source book* [477], which covers a wide range of relevant subject areas. It is split into various sections on professional and clinical issues and clinical interest groups. The lack of subject index is a deficiency that should not detract from an excellent publication. *Physiotherapy in the community* [478], edited by A. Gibson, is a combination of a reference book and textbook. Each chapter, on topics such as mental illness and strokes, also includes a list of relevant addresses and legislation. The National Association of Health Authorities has produced the *NHS handbook* [479], which includes a section on physiotherapy staff levels and training. Practising UK physiotherapists are listed in the *Physiotherapists' Register* [480], produced and published by the Council for Professions Supplementary to Medicine (CPSM).

Out of the wide range of medical encyclopaedias and dictionaries available, the *Encyclopedia and dictionary of medicine, nursing and allied health* [134] is the most appropriate for physiotherapy. Twenty-two conditions, including asthma, rheumatoid arthritis and stroke, are covered in the *Disease data book* [481]. The rehabilitation of the condition is considered in each section. The annual *Research and Evaluation Register* [482], produced by the Chartered Society of Physiotherapy, provides a keyword and researcher index to physiotherapy research.

The joint American/British *New source book for the disabled* [158] covers a variety of topics, including aids and psychosocial issues. One reference book that concentrates on aids is the *Directory of aids for disabled and elderly people* [352]. The Disabled Living Foundation produces *Information Service Handbook* [156], a collection of 24 annually updated lists on subjects such as wheelchairs, communication and sport and physical recreation.

BIBLIOGRAPHIES

There are few bibliographies specifically covering physiotherapy. Lloyd and Fraser have written *The information needs of physiotherapists* [483], [484], which include a suggested list of physiotherapy books and journals for a small hospital. As part of its Specialized Bibliography series the National Library of Medicine has produced *Physical fitness and sports medicine* [485], which includes journal articles, books and audio-visual material. Historical references on hydrotherapy, electrotherapy and cryotherapy are included in Morton's *Medical bibliography* [114].

Despite this paucity of specialized titles physiotherapy is well covered in general bibliographies. *British Medicine* [487], a monthly publication, includes books, audio-visual material and forthcoming conferences in medicine. References on physiotherapy are listed under the heading 'Medical ancillary subjects'. In *Medical and Health Care Books and Serials in Print* [113] there is a section listing physical therapy textbooks. Journals are subsumed under the general heading 'Medical science'. The *British National Bibliography* [486] provides satisfactory coverage of new British physiotherapy textbooks. It is arranged in subject order using the Dewey Decimal Classification system with physiotherapy appearing under 615.82. There are further listings under electrotherapy, hydrotherapy, manipulation and traction.

The *Cumulative Index to Nursing and Allied Health Literature* [69] includes a section on newly published books. Each of the 24 lists in the *Information Service Handbook* [156] produced by the Disabled Living Foundation details books, journal articles and reports on that specific area.

BOOKS

The importance of *Physiotherapy in medical conditions* by Joan Cash as one of the first textbooks written for, and by, the physiotherapist has already been described. From this original title has emerged *Cash's Textbook of chest, heart and vascular disorders for physiotherapists* [488], *Cash's Textbook of general medical conditions for physiotherapists* [489], *Cash's Textbook of neurology for physiotherapists* [490] and *Cash's Textbook of orthopaedics and rheumatology for physiotherapists* [491]. Physiotherapy is now well served, with book titles being published in a range of countries, including Australia, Canada, the UK, the USA and the Federal Republic of Germany. Wherever possible the books described below include some contribution from a physiotherapist author.

Career guidance for those considering working in physiotherapy is provided by French's *A career in physiotherapy* [492]. Overviews of the work of the physiotherapist are covered in *Foundations for physical therapy in stroke rehabilitation* [493] by Carr and Shepherd, Downer's *Physical therapy procedures* [494] and also by Arnould-Taylor (a non-physiotherapist) in *The principles and practice of physical therapy* [495]. For final-year students occupied with revising, an appropriate text is *Aids to physiotherapy* [496]. For the increasing number of private practitioners, Buchele and Wynn-Williams [497] have provided a valuable management guide incorporating a comprehensive address list.

An in-depth understanding of human anatomy and physiology is essential for most applications of physiotherapy. The only title on anatomy and physiology written for and by a physiotherapist is Moffat's *Anatomy and physiology for physiotherapists* [498]. More detailed information can be found in *Gray's Anatomy* [499], now in its 36th edition.

It is now recognized that the physiotherapist has to be able to make clinical assessments and arrive at diagnoses, as opposed to functioning at a technician level. An introductory text has been provided by Parry, entitled *Physiotherapy assessment* [500]. A further title has been jointly written by Coates and King, *The patient assessment: a handbook for therapists* [502]. J. H. Cole [501] has written an introductory textbook on evaluating the strength and function of human body muscle. Accurate measurement has been identified in Rothstein's *Measurement in physical therapy* [503] as important in the professionalization of physiotherapy.

The subjects of inter-personal relationships and communication have generated publications specifically for the physiotherapist. As part of their Clinics in Physical Therapy series Churchill Livingstone have produced *Interpersonal relationships with patients: psychological aspects of clinical practice* [504], edited by O. D. Payton. The interrelationships between doctors, physiotherapists and patients have been investigated in Bourne's *Under the doctor* [505]. An overview of the behavioural sciences has been provided in *Psychology for physiotherapists* [506] by Dunkin. In mental health, case histories are used to illustrate *Physiotherapy in psychiatry* [507] by Mary Hare.

Electrotherapy, Exercise and Manipulation

The three areas electrotherapy, exercise and manipulation were stated by Williams[30] in 1986 to be still central to the physiotherapist. There are now a range of electrical treatments for the physiotherapist to choose from. A broad perspective has been provided by Forster and Palastanga's updating of *Clayton's Electrotherapy* [508]. Other books on this topic include *Principles and practice of electrotherapy* [509] and *Electrotherapy* [510]. Nikolova, the originator of interferential current therapy, has had his textbook translated into English [511]. Pain relief through transcutaneous electrical nerve stimulation (TENS) is the subject of Sjolund and Eriksson's book [512]. A work that concentrates on the physiotherapist's function in pain relief is *Pain: management and control in physiotherapy* [513].

In exercise therapy, Colson and Collison (a physiotherapist and a remedial gymnast) have written *Progressive exercise therapy in rehabilitation and physical education* [514]. The American perspective is given in Sullivan *et al.*, *An integrated approach to therapeutic exercise* [515].

There are a wide range of titles written on manipulation and mobilization. *Tidy's Massage and remedial exercises* [516] originally appeared in 1932. It was last updated in 1968 by Wale and is still available. A student text, *Massage for therapists* [517], has been written by Hollis but suffers from a limited bibliography. Other titles worth highlighting from the available range are Bourdillon and Day's *Spinal manipulation* [518], the Australian *Aspects of manipulative therapy* [519] and Maitland's *Vertebral manipulation* [520]. Different patient handling methods are described in *Illustrated transfer techniques for disabled people* [521], by Pelosi and Gleeson.

Normal Movement

A basic introductory text for students, entitled *Human movement* [522], has been written by Galley and Forster. Effective use of photographs and diagrams distinguishes *Understanding the scientific basis of human movement* [523]. A broad overview is provided in J. H. Carr's *Movement science* [524].

Life Continuum

The physiotherapist has a role at various stages of human development. Literature has started to emerge that examines the physiotherapist's role in obstretrics. McKenna has edited the title *Obstetrics and gynaecology* [525] in Churchill Livingstone's International Perspectives in Physical Therapy series.

Physiotherapy in paediatric practice [526], written in 1975, is still available, while Shepherd, an Australian physiotherapist, has written *Physiotherapy in paediatrics* [527]. A book examining the use of hydrotherapy in paediatrics has been written by Campion [528].

The physiotherapist has considerable involvement with the older patient and the 'ageing population'. Significant titles include Hawker's *The older patient and the role of the physiotherapist* [529], *Physical therapy of the geriatric patient* [530] and *Physiotherapy and the elderly patient* [531] by Wagstaff and Coakley.

Neurology

Physiotherapy is no longer concerned only with the movement problems resulting from neurological disorders. The emphasis has shifted to treating the whole person. *Cash's Textbook of neurology for physiotherapists* [490] takes this into account. The importance of seeing each patient as an individual is further reinforced in *Physiotherapy in disorders of the brain* [532] by Carr and Shepherd. Bethlem and Knobbout [533] have written a book concentrating on neuromuscular diseases, with the further-reading list being limited to books only.

Strokes have generated a considerable number of physiotherapy books. Johnstone has written three titles on various aspects of the disorder: *Home care for the stroke patient* [376], *Restoration of motor function in the stroke patient* [377] and *The stroke patient* [378]. Further reading is restricted mainly to references from the journal *Physiotherapy* [460]. In contrast, a feature of Banks's *Stroke* [537] is the quality of its annotated bibliography. Another physiotherapy text is *A motor relearning programme for strokes* [538] by Carr and Shepherd.

Cardiopulmonary

Cash's Textbook of chest, heart and vascular disorders for physiotherapists [488] is now in its fourth edition and was developed from the cardiovascular chapters in *Physiotherapy in medical conditions*. This new edition includes a useful glossary and list of abbreviations. Another title with a considerable reputation is *The Brompton Hospital Guide to chest physiotherapy* [539] written by Gaskell. More substantial coverage is given in *Cardiopulmonary physical therapy* [540] and *Cardiac rehabilitation: exercise testing and prescription* [541]. An interdisciplinary approach is provided by Frownfelter's *Chest physical therapy and pulmonary rehabilitation* [542].

Orthopaedics

Downie has edited a further derivation from Cash's original textbook: *Cash's Textbook of orthopaedic and rheumatology for physiotherapists* [491]. Two physiotherapy textbooks examining amputation are *Physiotherapy for amputees: the Roehampton approach* [543] and *Physical therapy management of lower extremity amputations* [544]. On hand injuries, Salter has written *Hand injuries: a therapeutic approach* [545].

Physiotherapists are concerned with the range of sports injuries. An English translation has been made of *Physical therapy for sports* [546], edited by W. Kuprian. For the English reader a problem could be the further-reading list, which contains German language books and journals. A comprehensive textbook on both sports and orthopaedic physiotherapy has been edited by Gould and Davies [547].

There is also a variety of texts examining the physiotherapist's role with spinal injuries. The German publishers Springer-Verlag have published *Steps to follow: a guide to the treatment of hemiplegia* [548]. This is written by P. M. Davies and is based upon the concepts of K. and B. Bobath. Two further texts are Nixon's *Spinal cord injury: a guide to functional outcomes in physical therapy management* [549] and *Tetraplegia and paraplegia* [550].

For rheumatology, Hyde has written *Physiotherapy in rheumatology* [551]. *Rehabilitation in rheumatology* [345], by A. Clarke, is written for the health care team and includes a physiotherapy contribution.

Research

The increased emphasis on and awareness of research has resulted in texts being written specifically for the physiotherapist. A basic introduction to research for the occupational therapist and physiotherapist, *Research guidelines: a handbook for therapists* [184], has been written by Partridge and Barnitt. Payton has included an excellent chapter on information sources in *Research: the validation of clinical practice* [553]. A collection of articles on research from the journal *Physical Therapy* [465], entitled *Research: an anthology* [554], has been published by the American Physical Therapy Association. Another American title has been written by D. P. Currier: *Elements of research in physical therapy* [555].

REPORTS

The British government has produced various reports that examine the physiotherapist's function in health care. In 1951 the Cope report, *Report of the Committee on Medical Auxiliaries* [556], concluded that physiotherapy should be prescribed and directed by a doctor. The 1972 Tunbridge Report [433] reinforced these ideas about the dominance of the medical profession in the physiotherapist's work. The resulting disquiet was influential in the setting up of a working party under the chairmanship of E. L. Macmillan. The eventual report [434] suggested the need for more autonomy for the physiotherapist.

The value of physiotherapy in the community has generated three reports [557]-[559]. A fourth report on health information [560], under the chairmanship of Körner, addressed physiotherapy: paragraphs 4.12 to 4.13 investigated the routine collection of a minimum set of data to provide the basic information needed for effective management decisions.

Bibliographical details of theses and dissertations completed by practising physiotherapists are included in *Physical Therapy* [465] and *Physiotherapy* [460].

CONFERENCE PROCEEDINGS

Most of the professional physiotherapy associations throughout the world hold annual conferences. The South African Society of Physiotherapy published the proceedings from its 1983 meeting as a separate volume [561]. In most instances the proceedings are published in the professional journal of that particular country, for example [562]–[564]. The level of coverage varies from transcripts of presented papers to brief summaries of events.

Joint meetings between the UK Chartered Society of Physiotherapy and the Health Education Council [565] and Hospital Physicists' Association [566] have resulted in separate publications.

AUDIO-VISUAL MATERIALS

With the emphasis on procedural information in physiotherapy, audio-visual aids are important as an information source. In the United Kingdom, Graves Medical Audio-Visual Library produces tape–slide materials, teaching slide sets, audio cassettes and videos, and has also started producing computer software and video disks. It publishes an annual catalogue with quarterly updates. Included among its range of productions are the videos *Safe handling and lifting in hospital* [567] and [567a], and tape–slide presentations entitled the *Bobath approach to adult hemiplegia* [568] and *Physiotherapy for children with asthma* [569]. The other major producer of health-related audio-visual aids is Camera Talks [1318].

Details of recently produced audio-visual aids are also listed in *British Medicine* [487]. The BMA/BLITHE Film and Video Library have produced a list of health films and videos available for purchase or hire [570].

EXTERNAL ONLINE BIBLIOGRAPHICAL DATABASES AND CD-ROM

Van Camp and Seeley[29] have contributed a comprehensive chapter on health sciences databases to *Manual of online search strategies*. The online databases relevant to the physiotherapist correspond with hard copy equivalents. *DHSS-Data* is a combination of *Health Service Abstracts, Nursing Research Abstracts and Social Service Abstracts*. *EMBase* corresponds to *Excerpta Medica*. *CINAHL* is the online equivalent of *Cumulative Index to Nursing and Allied Health*, and *Medline* is a combination of *Index Medicus*, *Index to Dental Literature* and *International Nursing Index*. *DHSS-Data* [99] reflects the holdings of the UK government's Department of Health and Social Security Library. *EMBase* [100] has 300 000 references added annually from the 46 printed abstract bulletins.

In January 1988, *Medline* [101] included details of 5 459 000 bibliographical references from 1966 onwards. In contrast to *Index Medicus* [58], *Medline* also includes the abstracts to some references (59 per cent of the post-1984 references). *CINAHL* [97], while predominantly concerned with nursing, does include selected articles from 3200 journals listed in *Index Medicus*.

A major development has been the application of compact disk—read only memory (CD-ROM) technology in information dissemination. One 4.72 inch plastic disc can store the equivalent of 275 000 A4 pages. In order to undertake a search a microcomputer and a CD-ROM player are needed. This development is significant because it will allow the end-user to do the equivalent of an on-line search, but without the expense. Once the disks have been purchased there are no further costs. In a survey of CD-ROM users in a health sciences library, Glitz[15] noted that 83 per cent of the searchers found the system easy to use.

Medline [101] is available on CD-ROM and can be supplied by any of seven suppliers, each with its own different search software. The producers of *CINAHL* [97] made the database available in 1989 in Silverplatter format.

CLASSIFICATION SYSTEMS

Most health sciences libraries use either the National Library of Medicine (NLM) or the Dewey Decimal Classification schemes. NLM uses a notation of two letters followed by numbers, with systems (respiratory, cardiovascular, neurological, etc.) being used as a starting point. These are then subdivided by anatomy, physiology and pathology, resulting in, for example:

WG	Cardiovascular System
WG 200	Heart, general works
WG 201	Cardiovascular anatomy
WG 202	Cardiovascular physiology

Physiotherapy is classified at WB 460.

A development of the Dewey Decimal System, the Universal Decimal Classification (UDC), is also used for physiotherapy collections. All therapy is included at 615, with physiotherapy at 615.8. It is then further subdivided, with headings such as massage (615.82). In contrast to NLM, UDC uses disciplines such as anatomy, physiology and pathology as its basis:

61	Medicine
611	Anatomy
611.1	Cardiovascular anatomy
612	Physiology
612.1	Cardiovascular physiology
616	Pathology
616.1	Cardiovascular diseases

Some medical libraries are based upon the Bliss system, in which physiotherapy is represented by HNV.

OVERVIEW

There were significant developments in the 1980s in the provision of information and information services to the physiotherapist. The core journals have consolidated their positions and significant new periodicials have appeared. Secondary titles specifically covering physiotherapy are now in existence. Physiotherapists are increasingly writing textbooks for their fellow professionals.

It would be unrealistic to assume that physiotherapists in general have become more receptive to printed information. Grabois and Fuhrer's work investigating physiatrists' views on conducting research has already been mentioned.[16] They also ascertained the importance that practitioners placed on various information sources.[14] The first three sources in ranked order all related to personal sources (colleagues, meetings, etc.). Textbooks and the clinical literature were eighth and fourth respectively. It could be that the more student-centred approach to learning alluded to by Atkinson[4] will eventually improve practitioners' awareness.

References
1. American Physical Therapy Association (1988). Guidelines on critically considering research papers. *Physical Therapy*, **68** (4), 555–6.
2. Arnell, P. (1985). Awareness of and access to physiotherapy-related publications: a professional necessity. *Physiotherapy*, **71** (6), 271.
3. Arnell, P. (1986). Communication through publication: the role of reviewers. *Physiotherapy*, **72** (11), 530–3.
4. Atkinson, H. W. (1988). Heads in the clouds, feet on the ground. *Physiotherapy*, **74** (11), 542–7.
5. Bohannon, R. (1987). Core journals of physiotherapy. *Physiotherapy Practice*, **3** (4), 126–8.
6. Bohannon, R. (1988). How to find relevant references for a publication. *Physiotherapy Practice*, **4** (1), 41–4.
7. Bohannon, R. W. and Gibson, D. F. (1986). Citation analysis of *Physical Therapy*. *Physical Therapy*, **66** (4), 540–1.
8. Bunch, A. J. (1980). Using libraries. *Physiotherapy*, **66** (10), 337–9.
9. Currier, D. P. (1984). *Elements of research in physical therapy*, 2nd ed. Baltimore, MD: Williams & Wilkins, pp. 34–50.
10. Dean, E. (1985). *Physiotherapy Canada* survey (1973–1982): trends to research. *Physiotherapy Canada*, **37** (3), 158–61.
11. Dean, E. and Davies, J. (1986). Frequency of citation and reputational assessment of contributors in physical therapy. *Physical Therapy*, **66** (6), 961–6.
12. Domholdt, E. A. and Malone, T. R. (1985). Evaluating research literature:

the educated clinician. *Physical Therapy*, **65** (4), 487–91.

13. Dyer, L. E. (1982). Professional development. *Physiotherapy*, **68** (12), 390–3.
14. Fuhrer, M. J. and Grabois, M. (1988). Information sources that influence physiatrists' adoption of new clinical practices. *Archives of Physical Medicine and Rehabilitation*, **69** (3), 167–9.
15. Glitz, B. (1988). Testing the new technology: *MEDLINE* on CD-ROM in an academic health sciences library. *Special Libraries*, **79** (1), 28–33.
16. Grabois, M. and Fuhrer, M. J. (1988). Physiatrists' views on research. *American Journal of Physical Medicine and Rehabilitation*, **67** (4), 171–4.
17. Harrison, M. (1987). Conspectus '87. *Physiotherapy*, **73** (12), 640–7.
18. Jaeggin, R. B. (1988). Disability Resource Library Network. *Bibliotheca Medica Canada*, **9** (3), 155–7.
19. Jones, J. and Rugg, L. A. (1987). An information system for physiotherapy. *Physiotherapy*, **73** (10), 526–30.
20. Nunley, R. L. (1987). Physical therapy for the twenty first century: rationale and recommendations for educational change. *Proceedings of the Tenth International Congress of the World Confederation for Physical Therapy*, Sydney, 17–22 May, pp. 76–80.
21. Parry, A. (1987). Guide lines to appraising research papers in journals. *Physiotherapy*, **73** (7), 375–8.
22. Peat, M. (1981). Physiotherapy: art or science? *Physiotherapy Canada*, **33** (3), 170–6.
23. The practice of physiotherapy (1988). *Physiotherapy*, **74** (8), 356–8.
24. Ramsden, E. (1987). Physical therapy in the United States of America. *Physiotherapy Practice*, **3** (4), 131–5.
25. Roberts, D. (1986). *CATS*: a new information service in physiotherapy. *Physiotherapy*, **72** (11), 533–5.
26. Rothstein, J. M. (1989). Clinical literature. *Physical Therapy*, **69** (11), 895–6.
27. Simon, T. and Jones, R. (1987). Information systems, resource management and physiotherapy. *Physiotherapy*, **73** (10), 522–5.
28. Stewart, D. W. C. (1984). Using medical libraries. In Downie, P. A. (ed.), *Cash's Textbook of general of general medical and surgical conditions for physiotherapists*. London: Faber & Faber, pp. 15–24.
29. Van Camp, A. J. and Seeley, C. (1988). Health sciences. In Armstrong, C. J. and Large, J. A. Jr (eds), *Manual of online search strategies*. Aldershot: Gower.
30. Williams, J. I. (1986). Physiotherapy is handling. *Physiotherapy*, **72** (2), 66–70.
31. Williams, R. *et al.* (1987). Information searching in health care: a pilot study. *Physiotherapy Canada*, **39** (2), 102–9.

7 Dietetics

Cathy Hyland and Karen Hyland

INTRODUCTION

Dietetics is the science of nutrition and diet as applied to the feeding of groups and individuals in health and disease. Dietitians are primarily advisers and teachers at many levels, from individual clients to their fellow professionals and the general public.[9] Dietitians are graduate scientists who, in addition to providing a service, are actively involved in research to further the understanding of the role of nutrition in the aetiology and treatment of many diseases.

HISTORY AND DEVELOPMENT OF THE PROFESSION IN THE UK

The first dietetic department in Britain was established in Edinburgh in 1924, followed by the London Hospital in 1925. The first dietitians were nursing sisters, although the first graduate dietitians were recruited in 1928. The need for a professional association was soon recognized and the first discussion meeting was held in London in 1932. The inaugural meeting of the Executive Committee of the British Dietetic Association (BDA) took place in 1936, the constitution having been formed in January of that year, with the object of advancing the science and practice of dietetics and the education of persons engaged in the science.

The BDA has had a seat on the Professional and Technical Group 'A' of the Whitley Council since 1949, the first dietitian being Miss Betty Stanton, and in the 1960s Miss Gwen Powell was elected Chairman of the Staff Side of the Whitley

Council Professional and Technical Group 'A'. The Association has grown and developed because of the efforts of determined and dedicated dietitians. The practice of therapeutic dietetics has undergone major changes over the past 50 years. In 1961 dietetic practice was largely confined to diabetic and weight-reducing diets; since then there have been profound changes in medical practice that have highlighted and enhanced the expertise of the dietitian. Over the years British dietitians have progressed from special-diet kitchen duties to health education and community dietetics; participated in conferences and congresses, nutrition research and training programmes; and entered the world of industry, freelance and media work.

The first *History of the British Dietetic Association* [625] was published in 1961. It was written by Enid Hutchinson, who highlighted the energy and pioneering spirit of the first dietitians, who started a new profession in a branch of science that was developing. The second history[1] was written to celebrate its Golden Jubilee, and covers the years 1961 to 1986, during which period many decisions were taken to promote and support a variety of initiatives which have influenced change; for example, state registration, all graduate entry and the move towards a more independent, consultant status.

In 1960, the Professions Supplementary to Medicine Act [729] received the Royal Assent, permitting the establishment of a Council for the Professions Supplementary to Medicine (CPSM) to register all persons engaged in these professions. In April 1961 the first Registration Council and Boards were formed; the dietetic representative and alternate Members of the Council were Miss D. F. Hollingsworth and Miss B. J. Jamieson. The Dietitians' Board was set up to prepare and maintain a dietetics register, and registration for dietitians began in December 1962.

In 1961 the first Honorary Chairman of the British Dietetic Association was elected, Mrs E. Scott (1961–62). In 1964 the office of Honorary President was created, adding the strength of Sir Norman C. Wright, CB, to the association. The major reorganization of the National Health Service in 1974 created both an opportunity for dietitians to teach nutrition in the prevention of disease (community dietitians), and a developing role as District Health Authority nutrition and dietetics service managers (district dietitians). At the end of 1983, Her Majesty The Queen honoured the association by accepting an invitation to grant it her patronage.

EDUCATION AND TRAINING IN THE UK

Since 1985 dietetics training in the UK has become all-graduate. Entry to the various degree courses for dietitians requires a minimum of two 'A' level passes, or the equivalent Scottish Certificate of Education grades, including chemistry and another science subject.[7] Courses vary from first degrees to two-year postgraduate diplomas, and are listed in detail in Alexander's *Directory of schools of medicine and nursing* [199]. Once qualified, a dietitian can choose to work in the National Health Service, industry, education, the media or freelance.

Post-registration Training

Post-registration training opportunities are a fundamental part of the professional association's continuing education programme for its members. Training courses being successfully run are for mature returners, and for those wishing to specialize in paediatrics, renal disease, community health, mental health, geriatrics and clinical nutrition, and clinical supervisory skills.

The British Dietetic Association is now investigating the validation and accreditation of its post-registration courses. For the dietitian who wishes to attend non-BDA courses, some suitable national opportunities are: City and Guilds course 730, Further Education Teacher's Certificate; Health Education Teacher's Certificate; combined training programmes in computing at Salford University; District Health Authority training programmes.

In addition to formal postgraduate courses the BDA has continued to develop a programme of study meetings, to help fulfil the postgraduate training needs of members. Its Programmes Committee plans and arranges general meetings, study weekends and study conferences within the policy of the association. All courses are well attended and very successful, indicating that members need and appreciate the chance to update their knowledge in the company of colleagues. Study conferences have been held bi-annually and study weekends are combined with the annual general meeting. The association publishes the conference and study weekend proceedings. The post-registration opportunities up and down the country are varied and offer the enthusiastic dietitian an opportunity to find many resources to help him or her keep up to date.

THE BRITISH DIETETIC ASSOCIATION

In 1947 the British Dietetic Association was incorporated as a limited company under the terms of the Companies Act of 1929, and the Articles of Association were drawn up, which led to the creation of the Council as the governing body. The BDA became a listed trade union in July 1982, and in November 1982 professional insurance was included in the annual subscription for subsequent years. Formal election of the Industrial Relations Committee was held in 1985, the same year as the issue to members of a trades union 'rule book', the Code of Practice. The first Administrator, Mr John Grigg, was appointed on 1 February 1985, and in 1986 a computer system was installed to serve this professional organization.

In order to practise within the National Health Service, all dietitians (whether with British or foreign training) must be registered with the Council for Professions Supplementary to Medicine (CPSM). In order to retain state registration, membership must be renewed annually. It is not statutory to be a member of the

British Dietetic Association; however, membership entitles the individual to professional insurance, vacant-appointments lists, monthly newsletters and a quarterly magazine and journal. The *Newsletter* [576b] provides up-to-date information on such issues as current research, new literature, book reviews, exchanges of information and forthcoming events such as symposia, medical and professional conferences, multi-disciplinary courses and study days. The BDA publishes and circulates to its membership a calendar of national events and business or Council meetings.

Dietitians frequently work singly or in very small groups or departments, and therefore particularly need the support of a professional organization if they are not to feel isolated or out of date. The service is also of particular importance to the 'returner'. Several regional branches of the BDA were formed in 1952, to provide local forums where dietitians could meet to discuss BDA matters and topics of mutual interest. Branch meetings are a good opportunity to exchange information with colleagues and to listen to an invited speaker. The number of branches increased from seven to eleven in 1975. Each branch produces its own annual calendar of meetings.

The Publications and Public Relations Committee of the BDA initiates the publication of information and teaching aids in relevant areas of nutrition and dietetics. It acts as a link with other organizations and manufacturers concerned with nutrition and dietetics. It also reviews relevant articles and publications referred to the association, and reports back to Council. It provides copies of statements made to the press for publication in the *Newsletter*.

Dietetics was the first of the professions supplementary to medicine to have an Adviser at the Department of Health and Social Security when in 1972 a full-time Dietetics Adviser was appointed to the Catering and Dietetics Branch.

The BDA is a member of the European Federation of the Association of Dietitians. British dietitians often travel abroad to work or for research. The European Community allows the free exchange of personnel between EC countries, but language is a barrier for many dietitians who would relish the experience of working in other European countries.

Specialist Dietetics Groups

During the past 15–20 years dietitians have developed individual professional areas of interest. As a result seven specialist groups have emerged within the British Dietetic Association to promote increased knowledge and expertise in these fields.

The oldest of these groups, the Renal Dialysis Group, was formed in 1972 to address the growing need for dietitians involved in renal dietetics to meet together for mutual support and education. The renal dietitian looks after the care of patients with kidney disorders; he or she must have general dietetics experience and preferably have attended a post-registration course organized by the Renal Dialysis Group of the BDA. The renal dietitian is expected to have a knowledge of renal physiology, medicine and related pharmacology, which enables him or her to modify dietary intakes as a result of the patient's biochemistry, clinical findings and drug treatment. The dietitian works as a necessary member of the renal dialysis team.[8]

In 1974 the Metabolic Research Group and Community Nutrition Group were formed. The Metabolic Research Group provides encouragement and a forum for dietitians undertaking research work to exchange ideas. To achieve credibility the profession must establish a sound scientific basis for dietetic practice. Dietitians use precise dietary measurements for the diagnosis of disease; in studying the relationship between diet and disease; to control the dietary variables when studying other physiological states; in monitoring the effectiveness of treatments; and in evaluating nutrition promotion programmes and the development of the dietetic profession.[5] Many of the members of the Community Nutrition Group are employed by District Health Authorities to work with their community agencies. The promotion of health and prevention of disease among the local population by improving nutrition and by increasing public awareness of the link between nutrition and health is their mutual aim.[3]

The Paediatric Group was formed in 1975 to promote normal growth and development in children, both in those with normal requirements and in those with special dietary needs.[10] The 1980s brought the emergence of three additional groups. The Parenteral and Enteral Special Interest Group dietitians are working specifically in the area of clinical nutrition by identifying and treating patients at risk of and with frank malnutrition.[2] Membership of the Nutrition Advisory Group for the Elderly is open to all dietitians who wish to develop special understanding and expertise for working with elderly people. Their aim is to eliminate malnutrition and improve nutritional awareness among the elderly and those who care for them.[6] The members of the Mental Health Group are aware of the direct effect of nutrition on brain function, and that malnutrition can adversely affect mental well-being. Poor mental health can affect the nutritional intake of individuals, causing a deterioration in nutritional status. These dietitians work with patients with either mental illness or mental handicap.[4]

At the time of writing two more interest groups have emerged – Liver and Gastroenterology. We await with interest their future development. All these groups meet twice yearly and are expected to produce fact sheets for the BDA general membership.

THE ROLE OF THE DIETITIAN

The role of the dietitian can be divided into five main areas: *Therapeutic* – giving specialist consultative services to medical and dental practitioners, teaching in hospitals and working in research, specialist and investigation units. *Prevention* – the major role of the community and/or district dietitian, in liaising

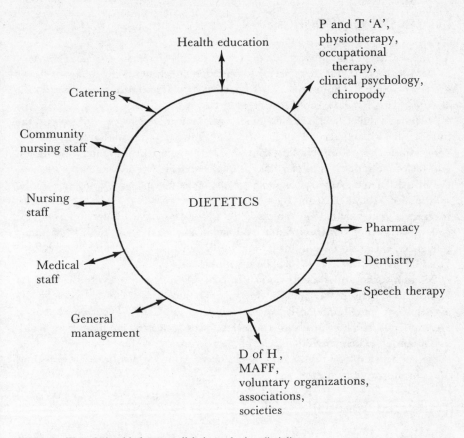

Figure 1   The relationship between dieletics and other disciplines

with health education departments, evaluating food research, and planning and participating in food surveys, research and health promotion projects. *Education* – teaching nutrition and dietetics to clients, student dietitians and students of many other disciplines, in hospital, community, university and college. *The media* – writing articles, books, papers; appearing in, advising on and writing for television and radio programmes. *Industry* – working as nutritional product advisers to food manufacturers.

The National Health Service is the largest UK employer of dietitians, but opportunities are increasing for dietitians to work in food manufacturing, pharmaceutical manufacturing and retailing, catering, food companies and retailers, the Department of Health (DoH) and the Ministry of Agriculture, Fisheries and Food (MAFF). This young profession is continuing to expand and develop to keep abreast of medical, science and technology advances, and to respond to the needs of its clients.

INFORMATION SOURCES

The profession has no single guide to literature and reference material. However, to find out about literature referring to nutrition and dietetics the following books are most useful: the annual *Willing's Press Guide* [57a] and *Medical and Health Care Books and Serials in Print*, published in alternate years [113].

Dietitians, allied health professionals and consumers can be confused by the number of available sources of nutrition information, and can have difficulty in determining the credibility of the sources. Dietitians use professional information and reference sources, i.e. periodicals, books and their professional association, the British Dietetic Association, whereas the consumer places importance on the information obtained from the media, i.e. the press, television and radio, magazines and health food outlets. Public libraries have limited information, generally classified under nutrition, health education and/or cookery. For detailed reference and up-to-date information, health sciences libraries and the King's Fund Centre Library [1249] will be the major centres.

Dietitians who undertake research projects will be registered with the Medical Research Council (MRC) and colleges through the CNAA; they are also encouraged to join the Metabolic Research Group of the BDA. The Department of Health sends Health Authorities copies of press releases, circulars and health memoranda, which are often relevant to nutrition, dietetics, cayering, food hygiene or technology. Quite often these need action by dietitians, caterers and other health professionals.

Translated Material

At local and district level, language is a barrier to communication, especially in multi-ethnic districts. In order to facilitate the understanding of dietetic advice and nutrition information, dietitians are forced to enlist the help (if available) of local translation services, such as the Linkworker scheme, the patient's relatives or staff.

Professionally prepared translated material is not abundant. The BDA has diabetic diet sheets in several translations, useful videos, photographs and slides of relevance to the dietetic needs of ethnic groups. The Health Education Authority has also published limited information leaflets and posters, and produced a video for dietitians to use in their work as health educators for organizations and individuals from ethnic groups. Commercially produced nutrition education literature is available from companies such as Heinz and Robinsons. Unfortunately, even these are still inadequate in meeting the requirements of our multi-ethnic population.

Publications of the British Dietetic Association

The official journal of the BDA was first published as a quarterly periodical from the spring of 1947 under the title of *Nutrition, Dietetics and Catering*. In 1972 the journal became a bi-monthly publication entitled *Nutrition*. In 1980 the BDA issued two titles published in alternate months, *Human Nutrition: Applied Nutrition* [591] and *Human Nutrition: Clinical Nutrition* [592], which combined in 1987 to form *European Journal of Clinical Nutrition* [579]. *Human Nutrition: Food Science and Nutrition* [593] was published for a shorter period, and continues as *Food Science and Nutrition* [588].

At the 1970 Annual General Meeting it was agreed that an additional monthly publication, a *Newsletter* [576b] would be produced for members (free of charge) as a vehicle for letters and exchange of information. This continues today as an essential part of the association's service to its members. Its first editor, from 1970 to 1975, was Miss Carol Bateman. Another service was provided for members in July 1981, with the publication of a quarterly magazine entitled *Adviser* [576a] and edited by Mr Neil Donnelly. This gives regular information to dietitians on products and short articles of interest.

The BDA has been involved in the production of a number of leaflets and pamphlets, either alone or in collaboration with other bodies. Today the association produces a selection of publications for the use of members: some of the current publications are listed in Part II [688]–[693].

September 1987 saw the launch of the new BDA *Manufactured Food Lists*, produced in collaboration with the Food and Drink Federation. These lists, of manufactured foods free from specific substances, have been compiled from a computer databank detailing several thousand food products that are free from ingredients to which certain individuals are known to be intolerant or sensitive. The databank was established with the full support of the Royal College of Physicians, the British Nutrition Foundation, the BDA and the food industry, together with leading agricultural and food research institutes. The databank is based at Leatherhead in Surrey, and access to it is available only through a state-registered dietitian or hospital physician. Not all food manufacturers have as yet participated in the databank, but they are being actively encouraged to do so.

References

1. Bateman, C. (1986). *The history of the British Dietetic Association, 1961–1986*. London: British Dietetic Association.
2. British Dietetic Association (1986). *Dietitians in clinical nutrition*. London: British Dietetic Association.
3. British Dietetic Association (1986). *Dietitians in the community*. London: British Dietetic Association.
4. British Dietetic Association (1986). *Dietitians in mental health*. London: British Dietetic Association.
5. British Dietetic Association (1988). *Dietitians in research*. London: British Dietetic Association.
6. British Dietetic Association (1988). *Dietitians working with the elderly*. London: British Dietetic Association.
7. British Dietetic Association (1988) *How to qualify as a dietitian*. London: British Dietetic Association.

8. British Dietetic Association (1988). *The renal dietitian*. London: British Dietetic Association.
9. British Dietetic Association (1988). *What dietitians are doing today*. London: British Dietetic Association.
10. British Dietetic Association (1986). *The work of paediatric dietitians*. London: British Dietetic Association.

8 Speech Therapy
Pat Munro

THE PROFESSION AND ITS HISTORY

The purpose of the profession of speech therapy is to identify and treat disorders of communication. It is the only profession to deal solely with these disorders, which are widespread and take many forms. Speech therapists assess and diagnose the disorders that affect a person's speech, and treat these disorders. As in other areas, a speech therapist's concern is also to research and illuminate the causes of disorders of communication, and to help develop an understanding of them.

The profession has been in existence as such only for a few decades. Disorders of speech were known about earlier and had been treated, principally by doctors. The development of oto-rhino-laryngology in Germany in the latter part of the nineteenth century had, as one outcome, the establishment of a professorship in Speech Pathology at the University of Berlin Medical School in 1900. At the same time the development of the new science of experimental phonetics was taking place in France, and the contribution it could make to the study of normal and disturbed speech was soon recognized. Stammering and deafness received early attention, and developments in neurology pointed up the role of the brain in speech impairment. The value of speech therapy became apparent in the early part of the twentieth century. World War I produced numbers of patients with head injuries that led to speech disorders.

In Britain the first speech clinic was established at St Bartholomew's Hospital in 1911, followed by another at St Thomas's Hospital. Their directors were teachers of voice and speech and drama. Other hospitals followed: Manchester started classes for children who stammered, and the London County Council started services in schools. These beginnings show how long-lasting was the debate into the question of whether speech therapists should work only within medicine, or whether their field should more properly be in education. In the later decades of the twentieth century this question is still a matter of discussion, argument and litigation. One of the problems speech therapists encounter is the ignorance of most people about the profession, many confusing it with the teaching of elocution. Gradually more and better publicity is helping to inform people of the true nature of their work.

The early history of the profession is covered well by M. Eldridge in her *History of the treatment of speech disorders* [827]. In the UK the organization of the profession took place in the 1920s and 1930s. Two associations were founded: one from the remedial section of the Association of Teachers of Speech and Drama, which became the Association of Speech Therapists in 1934; and the other the British Society of Speech Therapists, founded in 1935. Each of these had a syllabus and Board of Examiners, which conducted examinations and awarded diplomas. They amalgamated in 1945 under the title of the College of Speech Therapists, which is still the professional association for speech therapists. Although it no longer holds its own examinations or awards diplomas, it issues certificates to practise, which speech therapists are legally required to hold.

Speech therapists are employed mainly in the National Health Service, although some are employed in special schools or organizations or work in private practice. Those in the NHS may be in hospitals and/or community clinics, health centres, etc. Their salaries and conditions of service are determined by the Department of Health. The main government publication on speech therapy services is the Quirk Report [870], the outcome of an enquiry into the numbers required to treat speech-disordered people identified at the time. Reports on the numbers of speech-disordered people have followed over the years, but there has been no other major government report.

EDUCATION

The teaching of speech therapy is now conducted in universities and polytechnics as an all-graduate profession. There are currently 17 establishments that run degree courses leading to the qualification of speech therapist. In addition there are postgraduate courses available at several of these training establishments leading to Master's degrees. Several places also offer short-course programmes in individual subjects of interest to professionals in speech therapy and allied professions.

The International Association of Logopaedics and Phoniatrics was founded in 1924. The USA and most Commonwealth countries have professional associations, as do many other countries. In the UK there are many societies, mainly charities, interested in speech disorders. In addition there are societies for different disorders that have connections with speech, such as the Spastics Society and the Parkinson's Disease Society. Many of these organizations are publishers of journals, books and pamphlets of interest to the profesion, and are listed in Part III.

THE LITERATURE

The history of the literature of speech therapy is discussed in Rieber and Froeschels's 'An historical review of the European literature in speech pathology' and in West's 'An historical review of the American literature in speech pathology', two chapters in *Speech pathology: an international study of the science*, edited by Rieber and Brubaker [824], which are of interest. This book also contains chapters on current trends in various countries, including 'Speech pathology in Great Britain', by van Thal.

There are no major guides to the literature. A dip into *A medical bibliography (Garrison and Morton)* [114] for books on the history of speech disorders reveals that nearly all books are in French or German, reflecting the early discoveries in the field. One is driven to seeking out specialist bibliographies in various journals, some examples of which are given in the listings [796]–[798]; sadly these are soon out of date.

Abstracts and Indexes

Abstracts of the literature were covered well in *DSH Abstracts* [790], which is now discontinued. Sections of the literature are now covered in *Linguistics Abstracts* [792], *Linguistics and Language Behavior Abstracts* [793] and *Child Development Abstracts* [788].

The Current Awareness Topic Search (CATS) series from the British Library Medical Information Service, published monthly, is invaluable, but necessitates lengthy searches because of the absence of any cumulative indexes. The main titles in this field are *Hearing* [76] and *Language and Speech Disorders* [77].

In 1988 a new title, *Rehabilitation Index* [80], was started; this has an author and title index in each issue. Reflecting further the variety of subject matter contained in the literature, other current awareness services include those from the British Institute of Mental Handicap [324] and the Royal National Institute for the Deaf [795]. Journals that contain abstracts, such as *Developmental Medicine and Child Neurology* [789], are also useful sources.

Periodicals

The many journals [730]–[787] containing information of interest to speech therapists reflect the breadth and complexity of their subject interests. More peripheral titles, particularly in the field of psychology [764]–[769], occasionally have papers of interest in them. As with all applied sciences and branches of medicine, new information and ideas are always emerging and, in addition to journal articles, conference proceedings [859]–[863] are a way of keeping up to date.

Books

The variety of subjects of interest is illustrated in the lists of books [799]–[845] containing information vital to the study of speech therapy. The textbooks given are a select list, the study of which is essential to embrace fully the complexities of speech therapy. Speech disorders and language disorders, although not the same, have become almost interchangeable terms in titles of books and papers. Stammering and stuttering are different words for the same disorder, as are apraxia and dyspraxia, aphasia and dysphasia, etc. Literature on therapy procedures has long been available, principally from the USA. Over the past 10 years British books have considerably increased in number, and recently a series of such books has appeared from Winslow Press in their *Working with . . .* series [833]–[839].

TESTS AND ASSESSMENTS

Tests or assessments are tools used in speech therapy clinics to measure abilities and to diagnose disabilities; only a very few examples are listed [864]–[869]. They form an important element in the therapist's battery of working material. There are many on the market and the choice is varied, being dictated by needs and preference. Most are produced by commercial companies, the leading one in the UK being NFER-Nelson [1306], which also produces psychological and educational tests. There are also published programmes that therapists can use with their patients as part of their treatment. This type of material can be confusing to the lay person, as parts are often published as books that can be read in their own right as well as being instructions for the operation of the test. Examples include Goodglass and Kaplan (Boston) [866] and Crystal, Fletcher and Garman (LARSP) [868]. Some tests are restricted in their use, and readers are required to go on training courses before they can administer them. There are reference books that detail these tests and others, the chief one being *Mental Measurements Yearbook*, edited by O. K. Buros [864].

The Royal Association for Disability and Rehabilitation (RADAR) [1132] holds an exhibition of aids for the handicapped called NAIDEX each year; equipment used by the speech handicapped is included. Other equipment for use in clinics, such as word games for children, is produced by companies like Learning Development Aids of Wisbech [1301]. Their catalogues provide invaluable information of practical use to therapists.

The essential material used for testing the abilities of patients published by NFER-Nelson [1306] has already been mentioned; NFER is the National Foundation for Educational Research, and their catalogue is updated each year.

Information and advice is available at their headquarters and it is possible to inspect the tests there. A library of tests is also maintained at the Continuing Education Department of the National Hospitals College of Speech Sciences [1252].

LIBRARIES

The majority of training establishments (colleges offering courses that lead to a qualification in speech therapy) are part of a polytechnic or university, and the libraries serving these will have sections devoted to the relevant literature. The only one that has a separate specialist library is the National Hospitals College of Speech Sciences (NHCSS) [1252], which teaches a degree course in conjunction with University College London. The other major library is that at the Royal National Institute for the Deaf (RNID) [1262], which, although containing material principally on deafness and the deaf, has a considerable collection relevant to speech therapy. It offers a current awareness service in addition to a loan service, and is staffed by professional librarians. It has its own specialist classification scheme and an extensive catalogue. The RNID also runs courses and carries out research, and the library is open to anybody.

The libraries of the British Postgraduate Medical Federation Institutes (University of London), particularly of Neurology [1247] and Laryngology and Otology [1246], also hold relevant material. The library of the Whitefields Centre for special needs [1276] issues a regular bulletin containing recent lists of acquisitions and periodical articles. The NHCSS library issues an accessions list at two-monthly intervals.

9 Radiography, Diagnostic and Therapeutic

Linda Castleton and Mary Lovegrove

HISTORY

In 1897, Professor Silvanus Thompson wrote that the date of 8 November 1895 would forever be memorable in the history of science for the great discovery of X-rays by Professor William Conrad Roentgen in his physics laboratory at the University of Würzburg in Bavaria. These invisible rays penetrated cardboard, wood and cloth with ease and fell in shadows upon a luminescent screen. Metals such as copper, iron, lead, silver and gold were less penetrable, the densest being practically opaque. Strangest of all was when Roentgen interposed his hand between the source, a Crookes tube, and the luminescent cardboard and saw the bones of his living hand silhouetted upon the screen.

In 1902 Sir James Mackenzie Davidson reported that the greatest practical importance of X-rays was their utility in medicine and that the three prerequisites for making a radiograph – a vacuum, a source of electricity and a sensitive emulsion – were a scientific reality. The first two prerequisites were achieved by the Crookes tube designed in the 1870s and the third had been discovered two centuries earlier by J. H. Schulze, a German physician. Schulze, while experimenting with chalk and nitric acid, happened to use a solution of the acid in which he had previously dissolved silver. He observed that the white mixture turned black on exposure to sunlight and correctly attributed this change to the actinic effect on silver nitrate, a property still in use in radiography today.

The first permanent X-ray units were acquired and installed in the more famous London hospitals between February and June of 1896 and immediately put to clinical use. Some hospitals already possessed electro-therapeutic departments and, where they existed, these departments were extended to incorporate the X-ray unit. Diagnostic and therapeutic X-rays became an additional clinical service. Ernest Hamack and his three assistants, Reginald Blackall, Ernest Wilson and Harold Suggars, were the pioneer British radiographers. They were the first to be appointed 'X-ray operators', the first to receive radiation injuries and the first to die of X-ray-induced cancer. Suggars and Blackall were less severely affected and continued to work for a decade or more, and both were involved in the establishment of the Society of Radiographers, which was registered as a limited company on 6 August 1920.

SOCIETY OF RADIOGRAPHERS

The role of the Society of Radiographers was to promote science and to regulate the practice of radiography. The importance of protection was not recognized until later, when in 1929 the international recommendations for X-ray and radium protection were issued on the insistence of the British Committee at the International Congress of Radiology held in Stockholm in 1928. The first diploma examination for entry to the society was held in January 1922. One of the 20 to pass the examination was Miss K. C. Clark, the first lady president and author of the first major British work on basic radiographic positioning.

In 1926, the Society of Radiographers became affiliated to the British Institute of Radiologists, and University College Hospital prepared a scheme of training, which was formalized in 1931. In the early 1930s, branches of the society were formed in South Africa and affiliation was sought from Australia. This was the

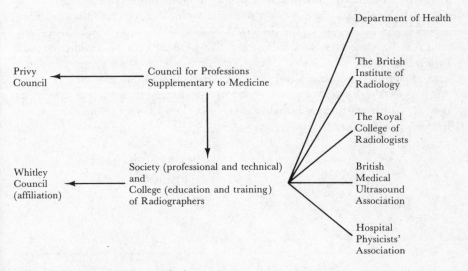

Figure 2   The structure of the profession

beginning of the International Society of Radiographers and Radiological Technicians.

DIAGNOSIS AND THERAPY

There are two types of radiographer: the diagnostic radiographer, who is responsible for producing the images and, in the case of medical ultrasound, often has the additional responsibility of writing reports; and the radiotherapy radiographer, who administers the radiation for treatment. The UK currently has two distinct but equal training programmes sharing a common core; one for diagnostic radiography and one for therapy. The training of radiographers is currently undergoing a major change towards degree entry for the whole profession; this change should be complete by 1991.

Diagnostic radiographers are employed in imaging departments, which are continually developing and expanding as new techniques are discovered and adapted for medical use. Since 1973, when the first computerized tomography unit was installed, there have been other major developments: medical ultrasound and associated Doppler techniques, sophisticated interventional angiography and, more recently, nuclear magnetic resonance.

Therapeutic radiographers are responsible for the planning and application of ionizing radiations for the purpose of treating disease, most often cancer. The methods of application available are far more varied than those outside the profession realize. Treatments may utilize externally or internally located sources of radiation and may involve any one of a range of radiations, e.g. X-rays, gamma rays, or particle beams.

The treatments are initially prescribed by a radiotherapist (a specially trained medical practitioner) but it is the radiographer who accepts responsibility for the accurate administration of the prescription and care of the patient throughout what may be a lengthy course of treatment. To fulfil their objectives and maintain their required role, therapeutic radiographers must develop expertise in all related areas, including localization and planning as well as application of the treatment. They must also have expert knowledge of the characteristics of the conditions treated, which are primarily malignant, hence the inclusion of oncology in the training programme.

PART II

Bibliographical Listing of Sources of Information

1 General Sources of Information

John Hewlett and David Roberts

USING LIBRARIES AND LITERATURE

1 Smith, B. (1986). *Sources of information on remedial health*. Coventry: Lanchester Polytechnic. 80 pp.
Very useful basic guide for physiotherapists and occupational therapists; discusses some 170 information sources and 20 relevant databases; bibliography of some 550 items.

2 Cook, A., Bailey, P. and **Ramsay, A.** (1981). *Health studies: a guide to the sources of information*. Newcastle upon Tyne: Newcastle upon Tyne Polytechnic. 109 pp.
For nurses, health visitors, physiotherapists and occupational therapists; outlines how to find information in health studies and the literature; exercises and answers; bibliography of some 300 items.

3 Dale, S. (1983). *The handicapped person in the community: guide to using the literature*. Milton Keynes: Open University E.E. Course E241.
Useful guide to literature on disability awareness.

4 Jenkins, S. (1987). *Medical libraries: a user guide*. London: BMA. 110 pp.
Brief guide aimed at medical staff and students; chapters include Availability of (medical) libraries, Finding your way around, The medical literature, Computer searches. Reviewed in *Health Libraries Review*, 1989, **6** (1), 56–9.

5   Morton, L. T. and **Wright, D. J.** (1990). *How to use a medical library*. 8th ed. London: Clive Bingley. 96 pp.
Useful guide for medical staff, with general applications.

6   Strickland-Hodge, B. and **Allan, B.** (1986). *Medical information: a profile*. London: Mansell. 145 pp.
For the medical reader; covers Printed sources, Online information retrieval, Organizations [including libraries] and people, Search strategy, Case studies and Organizing medical information.

6a   Livesey, B. and **Strickland-Hodge, B.** (1989). *How to search the medical sources*. Aldershot: Gower. 119 pp.
For the medical and pharmaceutical reader: limited in its scope (e.g. only three dictionaries).

7   Welch, J. and **King, T. A.** (1985). *Searching the medical literature: a guide to published and online sources*. London: Chapman & Hall. 128 pp.
Particularly useful on searching the periodical literature, drug information and statistical information; includes background reading and a section on reference books; for the medical reader. Reviewed in *Health Libraries Review*, 1986, **3** (2), 148–9.

8   British Medical Journal (1985). *How to do it*. 2nd ed. London: BMJ. 266 pp.
Brief practical chapters on many aspects of medical work, with some particularly useful for allied health staff. Reviewed in *Health Libraries Review*, 1985, **2** (4), 225–6.

9   British Medical Journal (1987). *How to do it 2*. London: BMJ. 208 pp.
As [8].

10   Binger, J. L. and **Jensen, L. M.** (1980). *Lippincott's Guide to nursing literature: a handbook for students, writers and researchers*. Philadelphia: J. B. Lippincott. 303 pp.
Very useful guide for nurses, with applications for allied health workers; good on keeping updated, reference sources of all kinds and (US) libraries.

FINDING A LIBRARY

11   Linton, W. D., compiler (1986). *Directory of medical and health care libraries in the UK and Republic of Ireland*. 6th ed. London: Library Association for the Medical Health and Welfare Libraries Group. New ed. expected 1990.
Lists 604 UK and Irish health care libraries, by location, with indexes by personal

name, establishment name and county; not good for special collections within general polytechnic or university libraries. Reviewed in *Health Libraries Review*, 1986, *3* (4), 244.

12   Heap, V. (1982). *Sources of information for therapists: a guide to the availability of library facilities*. Canterbury: University of Kent, Health Services Research Unit. 60 pp.
Good list of postgraduate medical centres, but ignores college, polytechnic or university libraries.

13   Codlin, E. M., ed. (1984). *Aslib directory of information sources in the UK*. 5th ed. Vol. 2, *Social sciences, medicine and the humanities*. London: Aslib. 1000 pp.
Lists some 3500 information sources of all kinds, with or without libraries; detailed indexes.

14   Medical Library Association (1979). *Directory of health sciences libraries*. Chicago, IL: Medical Library Association.
Brief directory of libraries; Backus's *Medical and health information directory* [152], vol. 2, contains newer information and a wider range of libraries.

15   Jaeggin, R. B. (1988). Disability resource library network. *Bibliotheca Medica Canadiana*, *9* (3), 155–7.

GENERAL INFORMATION SOURCES

16   Walford, A. J. *Guide to reference materials*. London: Library Association.
  Vol. 1. *Science and technology*. 4th ed. (1980). 697 pp.
  Vol. 2. *Social and historical sciences, philosophy and religion*. 4th ed. (1982). 723 pp.
  Vol. 3. *Generalities, the arts, languages and literature*. 4th ed. (1987). 872 pp.
A good guide to general reference sources, but does not cover the subject in great depth.

17   Sheehy, E. P. (1986). *Guide to reference books*. 10th ed. Chicago: American Library Association. 1560 pp.
As [16]; contains 28 pages on medical and health sciences, mostly general medical with some nursing, nutrition and pharmacology.

HEALTH CARE INFORMATION SOURCES

18   Brandon, A. N. and **Hill, D. R.** (1988). Selected list of books and journals in allied health sciences. *Bulletin of the Medical Library Association*, *76* (4), 346–67.

Standard American list, prepared for the Medical Library Association; no chiropody or speech therapy.

19   Brandon, A. N. and **Hill, D. R.** (1986). Selected list of books and journals in allied health sciences. *Bulletin of the Medical Library Association*, **74** (4), 353–74.

20   Brandon, A. N. and **Hill, D. R.** (1984). Selected list of books and journals in allied health sciences. *Bulletin of the Medical Library Association*, **72** (4), 373–91.

21   Chen, C.-C. (1981). *Health sciences information sources*. Cambridge, MA: MIT Press. 767 pp.
Has 4000 references with a strong medical emphasis; arranged by type of material, subdivided by clinical subject, e.g. Physical medicine and rehabilitation; good author and title indexes; no subject index.

22   Gann, R. (1986). *Health information handbook: resources for self care*. Aldershot: Gower. 251 pp.
Discusses the UK situation, self-care abroad and starting a health information collection. Reviewed in *Health Libraries Review*, 1988, **5** (3), 199–200.

23   HMSO (1988). *Department of Health and Society Security*. London: HMSO. Sectional list no. 11. 33 pp.

24   HMSO (1989). *Medicine and health catalogue 1989/90*. London: HMSO. 74 pp.

25   HMSO (1987). *Office of Population Censuses and Surveys*. London: HMSO. Sectional list no. 56. 18 pp.

26   Kurian, G. T. (1988). *Global guide to medical information*. Amsterdam: Elsevier. 808 pp.
Arranged by type of information, subdivided by keywords (without cross-references); good index, but no chiropody, dietetics, podiatry or speech therapy.

27   A Major Report. Dallas, TX: Majors Scientific Books Inc. 4 pa.
Useful booksellers list, particularly for American allied health materials.

28   Morton, L. T. and **Godbolt, S.**, eds. (1983). *Information sources in the medical sciences*. 3rd ed. London: Butterworths. 544 pp.
The standard work on medical literature; omits nursing and most allied health subjects; includes some nutrition and dietetics.

29   Chitty, M. G. and **Schatz, N.** (1988). *Federal information sources in health and medicine: an annotated bibliography*. Westport, CT: Greenwood Press. 306 pp.

An invaluable reference tool which includes information on the USGPO and NTIS as well as subject bibliographies. Reviewed in *Medical Reference Services Quarterly*, 1989, **8** (2), 98–9.

29a   Perry-Holmes, C. (1984). Nursing and related health areas: sources in US government publications. *Reference Services Review*, **12** (1), 49–57.
Reviews American government directories, guides, bibliographies and statistical sources in health care, particularly nursing.

30   Roper, F. W. and **Boorkman, J. A.** (1984). *Introduction to reference sources in the health sciences*. 2nd ed. Chicago: Medical Library Association. 302 pp.

31   Self, P. C. (1984). *Physical disability: an annotated literature guide*. Basel: Marcel Dekker. 474 pp.
A comprehensive survey of over 1000 works, all carefully evaluated. Reviewed in *Health Libraries Review*, 1986, **3** (2), 146–7.

PERIODICALS

32   *ADTA Newsletter*. Columbia, MD: American Dance Therapy Association. 6 pa. 1967–.

33   *American Archives of Rehabilitation Therapy*. North Little Rock, AR: American Association for Rehabilitation Therapy. 3 pa. 1952–.

34   *American Corrective Therapy Journal*. Rosedale, NY: American Corrective Therapy Association. 6 pa. 1947–. Now *Clinical Kinesiology*.

35   *American Journal of Art Therapy*. Northfield, VT: Norwich University for the American Art Therapy Association. 4 pa. 1961–.

36   *American Journal of Dance Therapy*. Columbia, MD: American Dance Therapy Association. 2 pa. 1977–.

37   *American Rehabilitation*. Washington, DC: USGPO for USA Rehabilitation Services Administration. 4 pa. 1975–.

38   *Behindertenzeitschrift*. Bonn: Rehabilitations-Verlag GmbH. 6 pa. 1964–.

39   *Behindertensport*. Zurich: Schweizerischer Verband für Behindertensport. 12 pa. 1962–.

40   *British Journal of Music Therapy*. London: British Society for Music Therapy. 3 pa. 1968–.

41   *Clinical Rehabilitation*. London: Edward Arnold for the Society for Research in Rehabilitation. 4 pa. 1987–. Includes *International Bibliographical Documentation on Rehabilitation*.
Covers a wide range of journals, but is essentially for keeping updated; retrospective searching is slow and limited.

42   *Information om Rehabilitering*. Bromma, Sweden: Handikappinstitutet. 8 pa. 1946–.

43   *Inscape: Journal of the British Association of Art Therapists*. London: BAAT. 2 pa.

44   *International Disability Studies*. London: Taylor & Francis. 4 pa. 1978–.

45   *International Journal of Rehabilitation Research*. Heidelberg: Edition Schindele. 4 pa. 1977–.
Included *International Bibliographical Documentation on Rehabilitation*, now published in *Clinical Rehabilitation* [41].

46   *Journal of Allied Health*. Washington, DC: American Society of Allied Health Professions (ASAHP). 4 pa. 1972–.
Includes *Index of Graduate Theses and Projects in Allied Health*. Annual, 1979–. Has included total of 1819 items, from 46 US institutions; 1987 issue listed 414 research items under 23 headings (except chiropody).

47   *Journal of Rehabilitation*. Alexandria, VA: National Rehabilitation Association. 4 pa. 1935–.

48   *Rehabilitación*. Madrid: Sociedad Española de Rehabilitación. 4 pa. 1967–.

49   *Die Rehabilitation*. Stuttgart: Thieme Verlag for Deutsches Vereinigung für die Rehabilitation-Behinderter. 4 pa. 1961–.

50   *Rehabilitation Digest*. Toronto: Canadian Rehabilitation Council for the Disabled. 4 pa. 1969–.

51   *Rehabilitation World: US Journal of International News and Information*. New York, NY: Rehabilitation International USA. 4 pa. 1975–.

52   *Scandinavian Journal of Rehabilitation Medicine*. Stockholm: Almqvist & Wiksell International. 4 pa and supplements. 1969–.

53   *Therapy Weekly: The Newspaper for the Remedial Professions*. London: Macmillan Journals. 52 pa. 1974–.

54   *Trends*. Washington, DC: American Society of Allied Health Professions (ASAHP). 12 pa. 1969–.

PERIODICALS DIRECTORIES

55   *Keyword Index to Serial Titles, KIST*. Boston Spa: British Library. Microfiche, annual subscription, revised quarterly.
Contains some 420 000 titles, including 330 000 from the British Library; invaluable for tracing correct titles, or titles on a specific subject.

56   **National Library of Medicine**. *List of Journals Indexed in Index Medicus*. Washington, DC: NTIS. Hard copy, annual.
Contains limited information on about 3000 titles; listed by *Index Medicus* abbreviated title, full title, subject field, country of origin.

57   *Ulrich's International periodicals directory*. New York, NY: Bowker. Hard copy, alternate years. 3 volumes, 5580 pp. (1988). Microfiche, annual subscription, revised quarterly. CD-ROM, annual.
Invaluable for all periodicals information, giving the fullest details; indexes are accurate and up-to-date.

57a   *Willing's Press Guide: a guide to the press of the United Kingdom and the principal publications. . . .* East Grinstead: British Media Publications. Annual.
Brief guide to periodical publications of all kinds.

INDEXES, ABSTRACTS, CURRENT AWARENESS

58   *Index Medicus*. Washington, DC: USGPO. 12 pa, cumulated annually. 330 000 entries (1988).
Equivalent online database is *Medline* [101].

59   **National Library of Medicine**. *List of Serials Indexed for Online Users*. Washington, DC: NTIS. Annual.
Complete bibliographic information on serials in Medline including the backfiles to 1966; a single alphabetical listing by *Index Medicus* abbreviated title.

60   **National Library of Medicine**. *Medical Subject Headings (MeSH)*. Washington, DC: NTIS. Annual, issued with the January issue of *Index Medicus*.

61   National Library of Medicine. *Medical Subject Headings (MeSH): Annotated Alphabetic List*. Washington, DC: NTIS. Annual.
Alphabetical listing of about 16 000 terms and 77 subheadings with detailed annotations; each issue contains a list of new terms with definitions.

62   National Library of Medicine. *Medical Subject Headings (MeSH): Tree Structures*. Washington, DC: NTIS. Annual.
Hierarchical listing of *MeSH* terms.

63   National Library of Medicine. *Permuted Medical Subject Headings*. Washington, DC: NTIS. Annual.
Alphabetical list of all significant words appearing in *MeSH* terms followed by all *MeSH* terms in which that word appears.

64   Strickland-Hodge, B. (1986). *How to use Index Medicus and Excerpta Medica*. Aldershot: Gower. 60 pp.
Reviewed in *Health Libraries Review*, 1987, **4** (1), 59.

65   *Excerpta Medica*. Amsterdam: Excerpta Medica. 44 sections each published separately, 8–12 pa; indexes cumulated annually.
Equivalent online database is *EMBase* [100].

66   Excerpta Medica. *List of Journals Abstracted*. Amsterdam: Elsevier Science Publishers. Annual.
Lists about 5000 titles.

67   Excerpta Medica (1984). *Guide to the classification and indexing system*. 2nd ed. Amsterdam: Elsevier Science Publishers.

68   Excerpta Medica (1988). *Emtree classification*. Amsterdam: Elsevier Science Publishers.

69   *Cumulative Index to Nursing and Allied Health Literature (CINAHL)*. Glendale, CA: CINAHL Corporation (formerly Glendale Adventist Medical Center). 6 pa; cumulated annually in one volume.
Equivalent online database is *CINAHL* [97].

70   Cumulative Index to Nursing and Allied Health Literature. *Subject heading list with online guide*. Glendale, CA: CINAHL Corporation. Annual.
Described by Fishel, C. C. *et al.* (1985). *CINAHL* list of subject headings. *Bulletin of the Medical Library Association*, **73** (2), 153–9.

71   *Health Service Abstracts*. London: HMSO for the Departments of Health and Social Security Library. Monthly, with annual cumulated index.
Equivalent online database is *DHSS-Data* [99].

72 *Nursing Research Abstracts*. London: HMSO for the Departments of Health and Social Security Library. Quarterly, with annual cumulated index.
Equivalent online database is *DHSS-Data* [99].

73 *Social Service Abstracts*. London: HMSO for the Departments of Health and Social Security Library. Monthly, with annual cumulated index. 235 citations (Dec. 1988).
Equivalent online database is *DHSS-Data* [99].

74 **Department of Health** (1987). *Union list of periodicals currently received in head-quarters libraries*. London: Department of Health.

75 **Department of Health and Social Security** (1984). *DHSS thesaurus/classification of the health and social services and social security*. London: DHSS.

76 *Hearing (CATS)*. Boston Spa: British Library, Medical Information Service. 12 pa.
Current lists of citations derived from SDIline, the current month of *Medline* [101].

77 *Language and Speech Disorders (CATS)*. Boston Spa: British Library, Medical Information Service. 12 pa.
As [76].

78 *Occupational Therapy Index*. Boston Spa: British Library, Medical Information Service. 12 pa.
Current lists of citations derived from the CATS database (British Library Medical Information Service), arranged in broad subject groups with author and subject indexes.

79 *Physiotherapy Index*. Boston Spa: British Library, Medical Information Service. 12 pa.
As [78].

80 *Rehabilitation Index*. Boston Spa: British Library, Medical Information Service. 12 pa.
As [78].

81 *Terminal Care Index*. Boston Spa: British Library, Medical Information Service. 12 pa.
As [78].

82 *Complementary Medicine Index*. Boston Spa: British Library, Medical Information Service. 12 pa.
As [78].

83 British Library, Medical Information Service. *Thesaurus for CATS database: alphabetic list*. Boston Spa: British Library. Annual.

84 British Library, Medical Information Service. *Thesaurus for CATS database: hierarchical list*. Boston Spa: British Library. Annual.

85 *Abstracts of Health Care Management Studies*. Ann Arbor, MI: Health Administration Press. Annual, 363 pp. (1987).
Informative abstracts, arranged by subject categories; fewer items covered than by [88].

86 *ASSIA, Applied Social Sciences Indexes and Abstracts*. London: Library Association. 6 pa. *c.* 1400 pp. (1988).
Lists contents of some 550 periodical titles by subject, including headings such as Mentally handicapped people, Mentally ill elderly people, National Health Service; good author index. Reviewed in *Health Libraries Review*, 1987, **4** (4), 269–71.

87 *HELMIS: Health Management Information Service*. Leeds: Nuffield Centre for Health Services Studies, University of Leeds.
Wide range of services, including current awareness bulletins, selective information dissemination and online database.

88 *Hospital Literature Index*. Chicago, IL: American Hospital Association (AHA). 4 pa, cumulated annually. 1957–. 646 pp. (1988).
Arranged by *MeSH* subjects from 1978; includes Recent acquisitions by Library of AHA, *c.* 850 titles (1987). Cumulation available on microform from University Microfilms.

89 *International Nursing Index*. New York, NY: American Journal of Nursing Co. 4 pa, cumulated annually.
Equivalent online database is *Medline* [101]. Coverage of nursing journals is wider than in *CINAHL* [69]; indexes 270 journal titles, plus selected references from 2500 more; arranged by *MeSH* subjects.

90 *Nursing Bibliography*. London: Royal College of Nursing. Monthly, cumulated annually.

91 *Nursing Bibliography cumulations*. London: Library Association.
        1959–1960, 1969, 132 pp.
        1961–1970, 1974, 236 pp.
        1971–1975, 1985, 368 pp.
        1976–1980, 1986, 406 pp.
Reviewed in *Health Libraries Review*, 1987, **4** (4), 271–2.

92 *Rehabilitation Bulletin*. Wakefield, W. Yorkshire: National Demonstration Centre, Pinderfield General Hospital. 12 pa.
Current lists of periodical citations, reports and other materials in rehabilitation and related areas.

93 *Rehabilitation Literature*. Chicago, IL: National Easter Seal Society, later National Society for Crippled Children and Adults. 6 pa. 1940–1986.
Contained review articles, abstracts and indexed items from a wide range of journals.

94 *Year Book of Rehabilitation*. Chicago, IL: Year Book Medical Publishers. Annual. 1938–51, 1986–.
Covers some 110 journals; arranged by subject, including Exercise, Prosthetics and orthotics, Cognitive–communicative rehabilitation.

ONLINE DATABASES

95 **Arthur, A.**, compiler (1989). *Quick guide to online commands*. 2nd ed. London: UKOLUG, Institute of Information Scientists.
A summary of various command procedures for about 14 database hosts, including BLAISE, Data-Star and Dialog.

96 **Farbey, R.** (1987). *Medical databases 1988*. London: Aslib. 88 pp.
Lists 120 databases on biomedicine, health care, hygiene and pharmacology; omits databases available as CD-ROM; useful lists of producers/suppliers/hosts and 35 recent references; no subject index. Reviewed in *Health Libraries Review*, 1988, **5** (2), 122.

97 *CINAHL (Cumulated Index to Nursing and Allied Health Literature)*. Glendale, CA: CINAHL Corporation.
Covers nursing, allied health and related topics; contains about 75 000 references, from 1983 to date, adding 2400 references in alternate months. Hosts are BRS, Data-Star, Dialog. Equivalent printed index is *Cumulated Index to Nursing and Allied Health Literature (CINAHL)* [69]. Described by Fishel, C. C. (1985). The Nursing and Allied Health (*CINAHL*) database. *Medical Reference Services Quarterly*, **4** (3), 1–16.

98 *Conference Proceedings Index*. Boston Spa: British Library.
220 000 references from 1964 to date; database of conference proceedings received at BL DSC, searchable by title keywords, etc. Equivalent printed index is *Index of Conference Proceedings* [119].

99 *DHSS-Data*. London: Departments of Health and Social Security.
About 70 000 references from 1983 to date, including periodical citations, reports

and other 'grey' literature, mainly in administration and socio-economic aspects of health care; adds 1200 references weekly. Hosts are Data-Star, Scicon. Equivalent printed abstracting journals are *Health Service Abstracts* [71], *Nursing Research Abstracts* [72] and *Social Service Abstracts* [73].

100   *EMBase*. Amsterdam: Excerpta Medica.
4 000 000 references, covering 1973 to date, adding 15 000 references weekly. Hosts are Data-Star, Dialog. Equivalent printed abstracting journals are *Excerpta Medica* titles [65].

101   *Medline*. Bethesda, MD: National Library of Medicine.
5 500 000 references, covering 1966 to date, adding 25 000 references monthly. Hosts are BLAISE, BRS, Data-Star, Dialog. Equivalent printed index journal is *Index Medicus* [58].

BIBLIOGRAPHIES

102   *Whitaker's Books in Print*. London: J. Whitaker & Sons. Hard copy, annual, 4 volumes, 7740 pp. (1988). Microfiche, annual subscription, monthly update. Lists 450 000 titles in print in the UK, 3000 titles due for publication (1989); 58 000 new titles; 12 500 publishers and address; usually full information.

103   *Books in Print*. New York, NY: Bowker. Hard copy, annual, 7 volumes, 12 000 pp. (1988/89). Hard copy, mid-year update, 2 volumes, *c*. 3900 pp. (1989). Hard copy, forthcoming books, 6 pa. Microfiche, annual subscription, quarterly update.
Lists 800 000 titles in print in the USA by author, title and subject.

104   *Books at Boston Spa (BABS)*. Boston Spa: British Library. Microfiche only, 6 pa.
Lists 250 000 books published since 1979, including those out of print, by author/editor and title.

105   *HMSO Annual Catalogue*. London: HMSO.
Lists British Government publications, but only those published by HMSO; compare [108]; arranged by issuing body, indexed by author/subject and ISBN. See also [23]–[25].

106   *HMSO Monthly Catalogue*. London: HMSO. 12 pa. Arranged as [105] and cumulated into [105].

107   *HMSO Daily List*. London: HMSO. Issued on weekdays only; posted daily or in weekly batches.

108 *British Official Publications Not Published by HMSO*. Cambridge: Chadwyck-Healey. Hard copy. 6 pa. cumulated annually.
Lists *c.* 10 000 publications a year, with a separate keyword index on microfiche, cumulated 6 pa.

109 *United Kingdom Official Publications (UKOP)*. London: HMSO and Chadwyck-Healey.
Catalogue on CD-ROM containing records from 1980; expected 1989; updated quarterly.

109a *United Kingdom Official Publications: a guide for users of UKOP* (1989). London: HMSO and Chadwyck-Healey.
Contains a useful brief outline of UK Government publishing.

110 **Richard, S.** (1984). *Directory of British official publications: a guide to sources*. 2nd ed. London: Mansell. 468 pp.

Medical bibliographies

111 *Health science books, 1876–1982* (1982). New York, NY: Bowker. 4 volumes, 4600 pp.
Cumulated version of *Medical and Health Care Books and Serials in Print* [113]; arranged by subject; indexed by author and title.

112 *Health Sciences Audiovisuals*. Washington, DC: USGPO for the National Library of Medicine. Microfiche: quarterly updates on annual subscription.
Lists all material published since 1975 in each update; full information; more useful than [115] because cumulated.

113 *Medical and Health Care Books and Serials in Print: an index to literature in the health sciences*. New York, NY: Bowker. Annual. 2 volumes, 2481 pp. (1988).
The standard regular medical bibliography; lists English language books in print in the USA by author, title and subject; includes periodicals listing by subject, omitting some English titles.

114 **Morton, L. T.** (1983). *A medical bibliography (Garrison and Morton): a check-list of texts illustrating the history of medicine*. 4th ed. Aldershot: Gower. 1000 pp.
The standard reference bibliography, particularly for historical sources; arranged by subject with detailed author and subject indexes. [143] and [145] also give references to historical sources.

115 *NLM Audiovisuals Catalog*. Washington, DC: USGPO for the National Library of Medicine. Hard copy, quarterly, cumulated annually.
New material only; compare [112].

116   *NLM Catalog* (1984). Washington, DC: USGPO for the National Library of Medicine.
Single publication of microfiche list of some 585 000 titles on 796 fiche; author/title and subject arrangement; full information.

117   *NLM Catalog supplements.* Washington, DC: USGPO for the National Library of Medicine. Microfiche, quarterly updates on annual subscription.
Lists all material published since 1984; full information; more useful than [118] because cumulated.

118   *NLM Current Catalog.* Washington, DC: USGPO for the National Library of Medicine. Hard copy, quarterly, cumulated annually.
New material only; compare [117].

CONFERENCES AND PROCEEDINGS

119   *Index of Conference Proceedings.* Boston Spa: British Library. Hard copy, monthly since 1966, cumulated annually 1974-. Cumulations, 1964-1973; 1974-1978; 1964-1981 (microfiche).
Lists a total of 220 000 references from 1964; adds about 18 000 titles annually; arranged by title keywords; full details. Equivalent online database is *Conference Proceedings Index* [98].

120   *Index to Scientific and Technical Proceedings.* Philadelphia, PA: Institute for Scientific Information. 12 pa. Cumulated annually.
Indexes 3600 conferences annually, some as periodical issues; arranged by 200 subject groups; indexed by subject, author/editor, sponsor, location; includes authors' addresses.

121   *Index to Social Sciences and Humanities Proceedings.* Philadelphia, PA: Institute for Scientific Information. 4 pa. Cumulated annually.
Indexes 900 conferences, 21 000 papers annually; arrangement as [120].

DICTIONARIES

121a   **Weller, B. F.** (1989). *Baillière's Encyclopaedic dictionary of nursing and health care.* London: Baillière Tindall. 1072 pp.
A new British dictionary covering health care terms.

122   *Blakiston's Gould medical dictionary* (1979). 4th ed. New York, NY: McGraw-Hill. 1828 pp.
Originally the *New medical dictionary*, by G. M. Gould, 1890; contains coloured anatomy illustrations.

122a *Churchill's Illustrated medical dictionary* (1989). Edinburgh: Churchill Livingstone. 2000 pp.

Almost 100 000 entries, including British and American spellings; new line drawings and coloured illustrations.

123 Clegg, J. (1980). *Dictionary of social services policy and practice.* London: Bedford Square Press and NCVO. 148 pp.

Contains short list of reports relevant to (health and) medical sciences.

124 *Concise medical dictionary* (1985). 2nd ed. Oxford: OUP. 677 pp.

Intended 'primarily for workers in the paramedical fields', including nurses; some illustrations; short but useful.

125 Council of Europe (1988). *Legislation on the rehabilitation of disabled people in thirteen member states.* 3rd ed. Strasbourg: Council of Europe. 280 pp.

126 Council of Europe (1985). *Rehabilitation of disabled persons: glossary and list of the principal terms.* 3rd ed. London: HMSO. 130 pp.

Useful guide to terminology.

127 Critchley, M. (1978). *Butterworth's Medical dictionary.* 2nd ed. London: Butterworth. 1974 pp.

The standard work for British medical terms; contains extensive anatomical nomenclature.

128 Dorland, W. A. N. (1988). *Dorland's Illustrated medical dictionary.* 27th ed. Philadelphia, PA: W. B. Saunders. 1920 pp.

1st ed., 1900; reliable American standard work, included in the list of standard works in the bibliography to *Medical Subject Headings* (*MeSH*) [60].

129 Dorland, W. A. N. (1982). *Dorland's Pocket medical dictionary.* 23rd ed. Philadelphia, PA: W. B. Saunders.

Abridged version of [128].

130 Lennox, B. and **Lennox, M. E.** (1986). *Heinemann Medical dictionary.* London: Heinemann. 611 pp.

131 Kamenetz, H. L. (1983). *Dictionary of rehabilitation medicine.* New York: Springer. 368 pp.

Particularly useful for physiotherapists and occupational therapists; abbreviations given meanings but often no further clarification.

132 Kamenetz, H. L. and **Kamenetz, G.** (1972). *English–French dictionary of physical medicine and rehabilitation.* Paris: Libraire Maloine. 93 pp.

Published with [133].

133   Kamenetz, H. L. and **Kamenetz, G.** (1972). *Dictionnaire français–anglais de médecine physique de rééducation et réadaptation fonctionelles*. Paris: Libraire Maloine. 85 pp.

134   Miller, B. F. and **Keane, C. B.** (1987). *Encyclopedia and dictionary of medicine, nursing and allied health*. 4th ed. Philadelphia, PA: W. B. Saunders. 1427 pp.
Broadly based, covering a wider range of subjects than usual medical dictionaries and including paramedical subjects; probably the most useful dictionary for allied health staff.

135   Glanze, W. D., ed. (1986). *Mosby's Medical and nursing dictionary*. 2nd ed. St Louis, MO: C. V. Mosby. 1484 pp.
Includes coloured anatomical illustrations; but often no references from British spellings to their American equivalents.

136   Schmidt, J. E. (1969). *Paramedical dictionary: a practical dictionary for the semi-medical and ancillary medical professions*. Springfield, IL: C. C. Thomas. 423 pp.

137   Stedman, T. L. (1982). *Stedman's Medical dictionary*. 24th ed. Baltimore, MD: Williams & Wilkins. 1678 pp.
1st ed., 1911; *c.* 100 000 entries; includes useful section on etymology.

138   Stedman, T. L. (1987). *Stedman's Pocket medical dictionary*. Baltimore, MD: Williams & Wilkins. 821 pp.
Abridged version of [137].

139   Davies, J. V. and **Jacob, J.** (1989). *Sweet & Maxwell's Encyclopaedia of health services and medical law*. London: Sweet & Maxwell. Loose-leaf, *c.* 4160 pp.
Contains all British statutes and statutory instruments covering the health services, and summaries of EC law; very well indexed; updated regularly as legislation is amended or passed.

140   Thomas, C. L., ed. (1989). *Taber's Cyclopedic medical dictionary*. 16th ed. Philadelphia, PA: F. A. Davis. 2450 pp.
1st ed., 1940; aimed primarily at nurses and allied health professionals; *c.* 47 000 entries.

141   Tver, D. F. and **Hunt, H. F.** (1986). *Encyclopedic dictionary of sports medicine*. New York, NY: Chapman & Hall. 232 pp. *c.* 5000 entries.

142   *Wiley International dictionary of medicine and biology* (1986). New York, NY: John Wiley. 3 volumes, 3200 pp.

Very broadly based, covering all biomedical sciences; probably not as useful as Miller and Keane [134] or the medical dictionaries.

EPONYMS, SYNDROMES AND NOMENCLATURE

143   **Jablonski, S.** (1990). *Dictionary of syndromes and eponymic diseases.* 2nd ed. Melbourne, FL: Krieger Publishing Co.
1st ed., 1969; arranged by name(s); includes original references.

144   **Lourie, J.** (1982). *Medical eponyms: who was Coude?* Tunbridge Wells, Kent: Pitman.
A useful list, although brief.

145   **Magalini, S. I.** and **Scrascia, E.** (1981). *Dictionary of medical syndromes.* 2nd ed. Philadelphia, PA: J. B. Lippincott. 956 pp.
Broader than Jablonski [143]; gives more detail.

146   **Firkin, B. G.** and **Whitworth, J. A.** (1987). *Dictionary of medical eponyms.* Carnforth, Lancs.: Parthenon Publishing Group. 592 pp.
Omits original references to syndromes; lists only 16 items in a bibliography.

147   **Davies, P. M.** (1985). *Medical terminology.* 4th ed. London: Heinemann. 400 pp.

148   **Rickards, R.** (1980). *Understanding medical terms: a self-instructional course.* Edinburgh: Churchill Livingstone.
Shows the structure of complex words and enables the user to break them down into component parts; gives origins from classical and other sources; explains the different origins of, for example, kidney, nephr- and ren-.

149   **Roberts, F.** (1971). *Medical terms: their origin and construction.* 5th ed. London: Heinemann. 102 pp.
Includes abbreviations for qualifications, societies and institutions, foreign and Latin terms; contains lists of source books and of 'the titles of the principal medical journals'; but omits some obvious allied health abbreviations.

150   **Steen, E. B.** (1978). *Abbreviations in medicine.* 4th ed. London: Baillière Tindall. 136 pp.

151   **Strauss, M. B.**, ed. (1968). *Familiar medical quotations.* London: Churchill. 968 pp.
The standard work, useful for apt quotations.

DIRECTORIES

152   Backus, K., ed. (1988). *Medical and health information directory*. 4th ed. Detroit, MI: Gale Research Co.
Vol. 1. *Organizations, agencies and institutions*. 1140 pp. Includes international (based in the USA), national and state associations; US medical and allied health schools, including podiatry, dietetics, occupational therapy, physical therapy, respiratory therapy and rehabilitation.
Vol. 2. *Publications, libraries and other information services*. 653 pp.
Includes international journals, abstracts and indexes, audio-visual programmes, computerized and online information services and US (medical) libraries.
Vol. 3. *Health services*. 767 pp.
Covers only USA health services.

153   Darnbrough, A. and **Kinrade, D.** (1988). *Directory for disabled people*. 5th ed. Cambridge: Woodhead-Faulkner. 356 pp.
Standard reference work for people with disabilities and their carers; includes wide range of information; good index.

154   *Directory of Hospitals*. Edinburgh: Churchill Livingstone. Annual. 430 pp. (1989).
Useful listing of all hospitals; indexed by health authority, by hospital type (including 220 'other') and location.

155   *Directory of independent hospitals and health services, 1988–1989*. (1988). Harlow, Essex: Longman. 720 pp.
Lists private hospitals, private screening clinics, private beds in NHS hospitals; private nursing homes; private homes; voluntary (charity-aided) homes; geographical arrangement in each section; indexed by name of institution.

156   Disabled Living Foundation. *Information Service Handbook*. London: Disabled Living Foundation.
Produced as 24 sections, each updated annually on a rolling bi-monthly programme; contains very wide range of information, including equipment, recent publications, addresses of suppliers and publishers, e.g. Section 6, *Leisure activities* lists 110 publications, 170 suppliers and 65 publishers.

157   *Equipment for the disabled*. Oxford: Nuffield Orthopaedic Centre. 12 sections, regularly updated.
Evaluates equipment, often by asking people with disabilities to test it and comment.

158   Hale, G., ed. (1983). *New source book for the disabled.* 2nd ed. London: Heinemann, 288 pp.
For the general reader; rather outdated (especially addresses) but still useful.

159   Hastings, M. R., ed. (1988). *Health and safety directory, 1988/89.* Brentford: Kluwer. 1036 pp.
Includes a bibliography, other sources of information, acronyms and abbreviations.

160   Henderson, G. P. and **Henderson, S. P. A.**, eds. (1988). *Directory of British associations and associations in Ireland.* 9th ed. Beckenham: CBD Research Ltd.
Standard guide to British associations; gives full information on *c.* 6000 societies and associations, arranged by title with a detailed subject index and cross-references.

161   *Hospitals and health service yearbook and directory of hospital suppliers.* London: Institute of Health Services Management. Annual. 982 pp. (1989).
Standard reference work on the NHS; contains information on health authorities and hospitals; list of statutory instruments, health circulars and health memoranda in force; bibliography on the NHS arranged by broad subjects (*c.* 800 items in 1987).

162   Keeble, U. (1979). *Aids and adaptations: a study of the administrative process by which social services departments help clients to receive aids and adaptations to their homes.* London: Bedford Square Press for the NCSS. 320 pp.

163   Kruzas, A. T., ed. (1983). *Encyclopedia of medical organizations and agencies.* Detroit, MI: Gale Research Co. 768 pp.

164   Robertson, S. (1988). *Disability rights handbook.* 13th ed. London: Disability Alliance.
Standard work, regularly updated. Covers rights, benefits and services, such as housing benefits, mobility allowances, practical help at home; useful address list.

165   *Social Services Yearbook.* Harlow: Longman. Annual. 806 pp. (1989/90).
Contains a wide range of information on all aspects of the social services.

166   Wasserman, P., ed. (1987). *Encyclopedia of health information sources.* Detroit, MI: Gale Research Co.
Broader based than [163]; *c.* 13 000 information sources, from 1980 onwards, largely US, in 450 subject divisions; some potential confusion, e.g. Audiology, Communication disorders, Deafness, Hearing disorders, Otorhinolaryngologic diseases, Otorhinolaryngologic surgery; no index.

167 *Who's who in rehabilitation: professionals and facilities* (1985). Chicago, IL: Marquis Who's Who. 429 pp.

168 Zeitak, G. and **Berman, F.** (1982). *Directory of international and national medical and related societies*. Oxford: PBX Informatics and Pergamon Press.

Listed by country; indexed by society title and by broad subject, e.g. Nutrition and dietetics 48 (but not the BDA); Podiatry 21; Rehabilitation (including occupational therapy and physiotherapy) 142.

GUIDES TO RESEARCH

Index of Graduate Theses and Projects in Allied Health, see *Journal of Allied Health* [46]

169 *Aslib Index to Theses Accepted for Higher Degrees by the Universities of Great Britain and Ireland and the Council for National Academic Awards*. London: Aslib. 2 pa. 1950-.

Indexed by author and selected specific subjects; does not include MA or MSc dissertations.

170 British Library (1987). *Current Research in Britain*. Boston Spa: British Library.

Biological sciences. 2 vols, 1143 pp.
Social sciences. 595 pp.

171 *Dissertation Abstracts International*. Ann Arbor, MI: University Microfilms International.

A. *Humanities and Social Sciences*. 12 pa. Also on microfiche, whole or in subject sections.

B. *Sciences and Engineering*. 12 pa. Also on microfiche, whole or in subject sections.

C. *European Dissertations*. 4 pa.

172 *Medical research centres: a world directory of organizations and programmes*. (1988). 8th ed. Harlow: Longman. 2 volumes, 1013 pp.

Useful international guide to general research areas, rather than detailed specific subjects.

173 *Medical research directory*. (1983). Chichester: John Wiley.

Useful but now outdated; may give general research areas, which can be followed up elsewhere.

GUIDES TO STATISTICS

174   Central Statistical Office. *Guide to Official Statistics*. London: HMSO. Alternate years. 192 pp. (1986).

175   Cowie, A. (1986). Medical statistical information: a guide to sources. *Health Libraries Review*, **3** (4), 203–21.

176   *Health and Personal Social Services Statistics for England*. London: HMSO. Annual. 175 pp. (1987).

177   Office of Population Censuses and Surveys. *OPCS Monitors*. London: OPCS. Various series, published at differing intervals, obtainable from OPCS, e.g. *Deaths by cause*, Ref. DH2, 4 pa; *Morbidity statistics from general practice*, Ref. MB5, occasional.

178   Office of Population Censuses and Surveys. *OPCS Reference Series*. London: HMSO. Various series, often cumulations of *OPCS Monitors*. Obtainable from HMSO, e.g. Series DH2, *Mortality statistics by cause*, annual; Series DH5, *Mortality statistics by area*, annual; Series MB4, *Hospital in-patient enquiry (HIPE), summary tables*, annual; *Main tables*, annual, on microfiche only.

179   Office of Population Censuses and Surveys. *OPCS Surveys of Disability in Great Britain*. London: HMSO. Irregular. 1988–.

180   *Scottish Health Statistics*. Edinburgh: Scottish Health Service Common Services Agency. Annual. 149 pp. (1986/87).

181   *Social Trends*. London: HMSO. Annual. 219 pp. (1988).

RESEARCH METHODS

182   Calnan, J. S. (1984). *Coping with research: the complete guide for beginners*. London: Heinemann. 158 pp.
Useful brief guide; can be read straight through.

183   Hawkins, C. and **Sorgi, M.**, eds. (1985). *Research: how to plan, speak and write about it*. Berlin: Springer-Verlag. 184 pp.

184   Partridge, C. and **Barnitt, R.** (1986). *Research guidelines: a handbook for therapists*. London: Heinemann. 120 pp.
Useful for all allied health staff; good glossary of terms.

185   **Reid, N. G.** and **Boore, J. R. P.** (1987). *Research methods and statistics in health care*. London: Edward Arnold.

How to do it: statistics

186   **Castle, W. M.** (1977). *Statistics in small doses*. 2nd ed. Edinburgh: Churchill Livingstone. 220 pp.

187   **Kirkwood, B. R.** (1988). *Essentials of medical statistics*. Oxford: Blackwell Scientific. 246 pp.

188   **Petrie, A.** (1978). *Lecture notes on medical statistics*. Oxford: Blackwell Scientific. 194 pp.

189   **Rowntree, D.** (1981). *Statistics without tears: a primer for non-mathematicians*. Harmondsworth: Penguin. 199 pp.

How to do it: writing and speaking

190   **American Physical Therapy Association** (1982). *Advice to authors: an anthology*. Alexandria, VA: APTA.

191   **American Physical Therapy Association** (1986). *Style manual*. 5th ed. Alexandria, VA: APTA. Revised and expanded index, 1988.

192   **Calnan, J. S.** and **Monks, B.** (1975). *How to speak and write: a practical guide for nurses*. London: Heinemann. 178 pp.

193   **Calnan, J. S.** and **Barabas, A.** (1981). *Speaking at medical meetings*. 2nd ed. London: Heinemann.
A useful guide to preparation of papers and audio-visual material, as well as public speaking.

194   **Cormack, D. F. S.** (1984). *Writing for nurses and allied professions*. Oxford: Blackwell Scientific. 184 pp.

195   **King Edward's Hospital Fund for London** (1982). *Preparing for publication: a style-book for authors, editors, compilers and typists*. 2nd ed. London: King's Fund. 62 pp.

196   **Kolin, P. C.** and **Kolin, J. L.** (1980). *Professional writing for nurses in education, practice and research*. St Louis, MO: C. V. Mosby. 218 pp.

197   **Mitchell, J.** (1974). *How to write reports*. Glasgow: Fontana/Collins. 157 pp.

198   Lock, S., ed. (1977). *Thorne's Better medical writing*. 2nd ed. Tunbridge Wells, Kent: Pitman Medical. 118 pp.

EDUCATION, CAREERS

199   Alexander, L., ed. (1983). *Directory of schools of medicine and nursing: British qualifications and training in medicine, dentistry, nursing and allied professions*. London: Kogan Page for International Hospitals Group. 712 pp.

200   Burrows, W. R. and **Hedrick, H. H.**, eds. *Allied Health Education Directory*. Chicago, IL: American Medical Association, Committee on Allied Health Education and Accreditation (CAHEA). Annual. 380 pp. (1988).

201   *Allied Health Education Newsletter*. Chicago, IL: American Medical Association, Committee on Allied Health Education and Accreditation (CAHEA). 6 pa.

202   Clark, R. (1989). *Careers in nursing and allied professions*. 4th ed. London: Kogan Page. 122 pp.

203   Ryckmans, E. (1983). *Working with disabled people*. London: Batsford. 96 pp.

204   Taylor, J. (1982). *Careers: working with the disabled*. London: Kogan Page. 104 pp.

MANAGEMENT AND ADMINISTRATION

205   Datafile 14, Paramedical (1987). *British Journal of Healthcare Computing*, **4** (5), 37–9.

206   Day, C. (1985). *From facts to figures*. London: King's Fund. 133 pp.

207   Goldstone, L. A. (1986). *Health and nursing management statistics*. Newcastle upon Tyne: Newcastle upon Tyne Polytechnic.

2 Chiropody
Erica South

PERIODICALS

208 *ACTUK Journal*. Penarth: Association of Chiropody Teachers in the United Kingdom. 4 pa.

209 *American Journal of Sports Medicine*. Baltimore, MD: Williams & Wilkins for the American Orthopaedic Society for Sports Medicine. 6 pa. 1972–.

210 Unused.

211 *British Journal of Podiatric Medicine and Surgery* (continuation of *Podiatry Association Journal*). London: Podiatry Association. 1989–.

212 *British Journal of Sports Medicine*. Mountsorrel, Leics.: British Association of Sport and Medicine. 4 pa. 1968–.

213 *Children's Foot Health Register*. London: Foot Health Council. Annual.

214 *The Chiropodist*. London: Society of Chiropodists. 12 pa. 1945–.

215 *Chiropody Review*. London: Institute of Chiropodists. 6 pa. 1938–.

216 *Clinical Biomechanics* (continuation of *British Osteopathic Journal*). Sevenoaks, Kent: John Wright. 6 pa. 1986–.

217 *Clinical Orthopaedics and Related Research.* Philadelphia, PA: J. B. Lippincott. 8 pa. 1953–.

218 *Clinics in Podiatric Medicine and Surgery* (continuation of *Clinics in Podiatry*). Philadelphia, PA: W. B. Saunders. 4 pa. 1984–.

219 *Foot and Ankle.* Baltimore, MD: Williams & Wilkins. 4 pa. 1984–.

220 *Journal of the American Podiatric Medical Association* (continuation of *Pedic Items*). Washington, DC: American Podiatric Medical Association. 12 pa. 1907–.
Contains a regular listing of recent periodical articles, compiled in co-operation with the National Library of Medicine, entitled *Bibliography of Podiatric Medicine and Surgery*.

221 *Journal of Biomechanics.* Oxford: Pergamon. 12 pa. 1968–.

222 *Journal of Bone and Joint Surgery*, American volumes. Boston, MA: Journal of Bone and Joint Surgery Inc. 8 pa. 1903–.

223 *Journal of Bone and Joint Surgery*, British volumes. Edinburgh: Churchill Livingstone. 5 pa. 1903–.

224 *Journal of Foot Surgery.* Baltimore, MD: Williams & Wilkins. 6 pa. 1962–.

225 *Practical Diabetes.* Petersfield, Hants.: Asgard Publishing. 6 pa. 1984–.

226 *SATRA Bulletin.* Kettering: Shoe and Allied Trades Research Association. 12 pa.

CURRENT AWARENESS SOURCES

Bibliography of Podiatric Medicine and Surgery, see *Journal of the American Podiatric Medical Association* [220].

227 *Diabetes Contents.* London: British Diabetic Association. 4 pa. 1987–.

228 *RECAL: Rehabilitation Engineering Current Awareness Listings.* Glasgow: University of Strathclyde, National Centre for Training and Education in Prosthetics and Orthotics. 24 pa.

229 *Sports Medicine Bulletin.* London: London Sports Medicine Institute and British Library Medical Information Service. 6 pa. 1987–.

230   *What to Read – Feet.* Guildford: South West Thames Regional Library and Information Service. 12 pa. 1987–.

ABSTRACTS

231   *Yearbook of Podiatric Medicine and Surgery.* Year Book Medical Publishers. Annual. 1985–.
Extremely useful abstracts and a good index of subjects and authors.

BOOKS

232   **American Academy of Orthopaedic Surgeons** (1985). *Atlas of orthotics.* 2nd ed. St Louis, MO: Mosby. 906 pp.

233   **American Academy of Orthopaedic Surgeons** (1972). *Joint motion.* 2nd ed. St Louis, MO: Mosby; and New York: Churchill Livingstone.
A sourcebook that should not be overlooked by students of biomechanics.

234   **Arthritis and Rheumatism Council** (1984). *Rheumatic diseases: collected reports 1959–83.* London: Arthritis and Rheumatism Council.

235   **Baden, H.P.** (1987). *Diseases of the hair and nails.* Chicago, IL: Year Book Medical Publishers. 313 pp.

236   **Baran, R.** and **Dawber, R.**, eds. (1984). *Diseases of the nails and their management.* Oxford: Blackwell. 318 pp.
The most important book on the nails, this is clear, well illustrated and has many references, both British and American.

237   **Beaven, D. W.** and **Brooks, S. E.** (1984). *A colour atlas of the nail in clinical diagnosis.* London: Wolfe Medical Publications. 250 pp.
An extremely good introduction to the subject; good illustrations and diagrams and adequate references.

238   **Brennan, M. A.**, ed. (1987). *Management of the diabetic foot.* Baltimore, MD: Williams & Wilkins.

239   **Charlesworth, F.** (1951). *Chiropodial orthopaedics.* Edinburgh: E. and S. Livingstone.

240   The diabetic foot. *Clinics in Podiatric Medicine and Surgery* (April 1987), 4 (2), whole issue.

241   Rheumatology. *Clinics in Podiatric Medicine and Surgery* (January 1988), **5** (1), whole issue.

242   Radiology of the foot and ankle. *Clinics in Podiatric Medicine and Surgery* (October 1988), **5** (4), whole issue.

243   Coates, T. T. (1983). *Practical orthotics for chiropodists*. London: Actinic Press. 127 pp.
Especially useful for information on padding and materials.

244   Connor, L., ed. (1986). *The foot in diabetes: proceedings of the 1st national conference on the diabetic foot*. Chichester: John Wiley.
Papers presented by the foremost researchers in the UK.

245   Ducroquet, R. J. and **Ducroquet, P.** (1968). *Walking and limping; a study of normal and pathological walking*. Philadelphia, PA: J. B. Lippincott.
The first book (after Muybridge) on gait using cinematographic methods to observe gait; excellent diagrams.

246   Durlacher, L. (1845). *Treatise on corns, bunions, the diseases of the nails and general management of the feet*. London: Simpkin Marshall.
This book can still be usefully read today – it has remained surprisingly up to date.

247   Faris, I. (1982). *The management of the diabetic foot*. Edinburgh: Churchill Livingstone. 132 pp.

248   Finch, J. D. (1984). *Aspects of the law affecting the paramedical professions*. London: Faber & Faber. 208 pp.

249   Goldsmith, L. A., ed. (1983). *Biochemistry and physiology of the skin*. Oxford: Oxford University Press. 2 volumes. 565 pp.
An authoritative review of biological properties and characteristics of the skin.

250   Harris, R. H. and **Beath, T.** (1947). *Army Foot Survey: investigation of foot ailments in Canadian soldiers*. Ottawa: National Research Council of Canada. NRC no. 1574.
A very important piece of research, constantly cited in current research papers.

251   Helal, B. and **Wilson, D.**, eds. (1988). *The foot*. Edinburgh: Churchill Livingstone. 2 volumes.

252   Helfand, A. E., ed. (1981). *Clinical podogeriatrics*. Baltimore, MD: Williams & Wilkins. 101 pp.

A practical book edited by a chiropodist who has sympathy with the elderly; many black-and-white illustrations.

253   Hughes, J. (1983). *Footwear and footcare for adults*. London: Disabled Living Foundation. 137 pp.
Aimed at nurses, social workers and community staff etc. who care for elderly people and disabled people.

254   Inman, V. T., Ralston, H. J. and **Todd, I.** (1981). *Human walking*. Baltimore, MD: Williams & Wilkins. 166 pp.

255   Jahss, M. H. (1982). *Disorders of the foot*. Philadelphia, PA: W. B. Saunders. 2 volumes, 946 and 724 pp.

256   Jarrett, A., ed. (1973–86). *Physiology and pathophysiology of the skin*. Orlando, FL: Academic Press. 9 volumes.
A magnificent work with many illustrations; each section is written by an expert and there are plenty of references to follow up.

257   Jones, F. Wood (1944). *Structure and function as seen in the foot*. London: Baillière, Tindall and Cox.
A classic, and still useful today.

258   Kelikian, H. (1965). *Hallux valgus, allied deformities of the foot and metatarsalgia*. Philadelphia, PA: W. B. Saunders.
This has many illustrations, X-rays and diagrams which make it of use still to those studying surgery of the foot.

259   Klenerman, L. (1983). *The foot and its disorders*. 2nd ed. Oxford: Blackwell. 465 pp.
Useful to students and trained chiropodists alike; clear and readable, with excellent chapters on radiology and on appliances.

260   Lake, N. (1935). *The foot*. London: Baillière, Tindall and Cox.

261   Le Rossignol, J. N. (1980). *Encyclopedia of materia medica and therapeutics for chiropodists*. London: Faber & Faber.

262   Levin, M. E. and **O'Neal, L. W.** (1988). *The diabetic foot*. 4th ed. St Louis, MO: C. V. Mosby.
A comprehensive work on the subject.

263   McCarthy, D. J. and **Montgomery, R.** (1986). *Podiatric dermatology*. Baltimore, MD: Williams & Wilkins. 257 pp.

264   McGlamry, E. D., ed. (1987). *Fundamentals of foot surgery*. Baltimore, MD:
Williams & Wilkins.
Useful to anyone working on the surgical sections 5 and 6 of the Society of
Chiropodists' Ambulatory Foot Surgery syllabus.

265   McMinn, R. M. H. (1984). *Colour atlas of foot and ankle anatomy*. London:
Wolfe Medical Publications. 96 pp.
A new edition is promised shortly, incorporating suggested improvements from
chiropodists.

266   Mann, R. A., ed. (1986). *Surgery of the foot*. 5th ed. St Louis, MO: C. V.
Mosby. 852 pp.
Formerly by Du Vries, this is written primarily for orthopaedic surgeons, but has
much of interest for chiropodists.

267   Mercado, O. A. (1985). *Atlas of podiatric anatomy*. 2nd ed. Oak Park, IL:
Carolando Press. 22 pp.
Clear and beautifully illustrated.

268   Millington, P. F. and **Wilkinson, R.** (1983). *The skin*. Cambridge:
Cambridge University Press. 224 pp.
A good introduction to the subject.

269   Morton, D. J. (1935). *The human foot: its evolution, physiology and functional
disorders*. New York, NY: Columbia University Press.

270   Munzenberg, K. J. (1985). *The orthopedic shoe*. Weinheim, FR Germany:
VCH Publishers.
Easy to read and understand and covers the whole subject comprehensively.

271   Neale, D. and **Adams, I.**, ed. (1989). *Common foot disorders*. 3rd ed.
Edinburgh: Churchill Livingstone. 339 pp.
The best British book for the student and the newly qualified chiropodist.

272   Pierre, M., ed. (1981). *The nail*. Edinburgh: Churchill Livingstone. 118
pp.
A useful introduction to this rather sparsely covered subject.

273   Read, P. J. (1978). *An introduction to therapeutics for chiropodists*. 2nd ed.
London: Actinic Press. 238 pp.
The best pharmaceutical book for chiropodists.

274   Redford, J. B., ed. (1986). *Orthotics etcetera*. 3rd ed. Baltimore, MD:
Williams & Wilkins. 848 pp.

275   Regnaud, B. (1986). *The foot: pathology, etiology, semiology, clinical investigation and therapy*. New York: Springer-Verlag. 705 pp.
Not written for chiropodists, but interesting and with many new ideas for treatment.

276   Root, M. L., Orien, W. P. and **Weed, J. H.** (1971). *Clinical biomechanics*. Vol. 1, *Biomechanical examination of the foot*. Vol. 2, *Normal and abnormal functions of the foot*. Los Angeles, CA: Clinical Biomechanics Corporation.
These two volumes are essential for the student of biomechanics: the text is detailed, well-researched and clear; the diagrams are easy to understand and reproduce; there are many references and a good index in Volume 2.

277   Runting, E. G. V. (1925). *Practical chiropody*. London: London Scientific Press.

278   Samitz, M. H. and **Dand, A. D.** (1981). *Cutaneous disorders of the lower extremities*. 2nd ed. Philadelphia, PA: J. B. Lippincott. 284 pp.

279   Samman, P. and **Fenton, D.** (1986). *The nails in disease*. 4th ed. London: Heinemann. 224 pp.
A good introduction to the subject, with more text but fewer illustrations than Beaven and Brooks's *Colour atlas of the nail in clinical diagnosis* [237].

280   Sarrafian, S. K. (1983). *Anatomy of the foot and ankle*. Philadelphia, PA: J. B. Lippincott. 434 pp.

281   Sgarlato, T. E., ed. (1984). *Compendium of podiatric biomechanics*. San Francisco, CA: California College of Podiatric Medicine.
An important text on the subject.

282   Tachdjian, M. O. (1985). *The child's foot*. Philadelphia, PA: W. B. Saunders. 800 pp.

283   Tax, H. R. (1980). *Podopediatrics*. 2nd ed. Baltimore, MD: Williams & Wilkins. 642 pp.
The best book so far on this subject; encyclopaedic in coverage, with a wealth of illustrations and many references.

284   Tillman, K. (1979). *The rheumatoid foot: diagnosis, pathomechanics and treatment*. New York, NY: Thieme.

285   Walker, W. F. (1980). *Colour atlas of peripheral vascular diseases*. London: Wolfe Medical Publications. 112 pp.
Useful for improving diagnostic skills; illustrations are clear and numerous.

286   Warfel, J. H. (1985). *The extremities: muscles and motor points*. 5th ed. Philadelphia, PA: Lea & Febiger. 120 pp.
Ideal for the student revising for examinations.

287   Weissman, S. D. (1983). *Radiology of the foot*. Baltimore, MD: Williams & Wilkins. 456 pp.
Covers a wide field, is fully illustrated and good in parts.

288   Williams, J. G. P. (1981). *A colour atlas of injury in sport*. London: Wolfe Medical Publications. 152 pp.
Like all the Wolfe colour atlases, it is beautifully illustrated and useful for diagnostic purposes.

289   Wu, K. K. (1986). *Surgery of the foot*. Philadelphia, PA: Lea & Febiger. 537 pp.

290   Yale, I. and **Yale, J.**, eds (1984). *The arthritic foot and related connective tissue disorders*. Baltimore, MD: Williams & Wilkins. 470 pp.

291   Yale, J. (1987). *Yale's Podiatric medicine*. 3rd ed. Baltimore, MD: Williams & Wilkins.

292   Zaias, N. (1980). *The nail in health and disease*. Lancaster: MTP Press. 260 pp.
The result of more than 20 years' research, this book goes into the pathology of the nail at great depth; fully referenced, copiously illustrated and well indexed.

REPORTS

293   Brodie, B. S. *et al.* (1988). Wessex feet: a Regional 'foot health survey'. *The Chiropodist*, **43** (8), 152–68.
A major study of the foot problems of the population of Wessex Regional Health Authority aged from 0 to 75 years.

294   Cartwright, A. and **Henderson, G.** (1986). *More trouble with feet: a survey of the foot problems and chiropody needs of the elderly*. London: HMSO.
An invaluable survey and containing much useful data, though not as clearly presented as one could wish.

295   Munro, A. (1973). *Children's footwear*; report of the Committee appointed by the Chancellor of the Exchequer. Cmnd 5243. London: HMSO.
Discusses the effect of ill-fitting shoes on children's feet, and makes recommendations to raise public awareness in this matter.

296   Clarke, M. (1969). *Trouble with feet*. London: G. Bell.
A study undertaken to estimate the troubles people have with their feet and how their needs are not being met.

297   Kemp, J. and **Winkler, J. T.** (1983). *Problems afoot: need and efficiency in footcare*. London: Disabled Living Foundation.
A major sociological study directly related to the chiropodial needs of people.

298   National Consumer Council (1981). *Bad fit, bad feet*. London: National Consumer Council.

299   Winder, R. (1970). Foot surveys published in *The Chiropodist*, 1946–69. *The Chiropodist*, **25**, 19–30.

STATISTICS

Health and Personal Social Services Statistics for England and Wales [176].

AUDIO-VISUAL MATERIAL

299a   Health Education Authority (1988). *Foot health: resource list.* . . . London: HEA. 11 pp.
A useful list, including print and non-print materials.

300   *Chiropodists don't just treat people* (1987). London: Society of Chiropodists. Video, for adults or teenagers. 20 minutes.

301   *Chiropody as a career* (1983). Northampton: Northampton Health Authority. Video, for adults or teenagers. 20 minutes.

302   *The five* (1970). London: BLITHE Audiovisual Library. Video, for 8–12-year-old girls. 7 minutes.

303   *Footcare for diabetics* (1983). Lipha Pharmaceuticals. Video, for students and adults. 18 minutes.

304   *Growing feet first* (1986). London: Foot Health Council. Video, for adults or teenagers. 20 minutes.

305   *The history of the foot*. Collagen Corporation, USA. Video, for adults.

306   *Sporting feet first*. (1986). London: Foot Health Council. Video, for adults or teenagers. 20 minutes.

307   *Working feet first* (1986). London: Foot Health Council. Video, for adults or teenagers. 20 minutes.

307a   *The foot*. Edinburgh: Churchill Livingstone. 4 pa. 1991–.
Aimed at chiropodists and orthopaedic specialists, with chiropodists on the editorial board.

307b   **Berquist, T. H.**, ed. (1988). *Radiology of the foot and ankle*. New York, NY: Raven Press.
This, though not aimed specifically at podiatrists, includes them in its target group. It is clearly an important book in its field, copiously illustrated with photographs and diagrams and with an excellent index.

307c   **Levy, L. A.** and **Hetherington, V. J.**, eds (1990). *Principles and practice of podiatric medicine*. Edinburgh: Churchill Livingstone.
This is a really comprehensive book, an excellent textbook for the four-year honours degree course and for the practising podiatrist. The authors of chapters are practising podiatrists and medical experts, all American except Dagnall, who writes on basic operative procedures.

3 Occupational Therapy

Margie Mellis

PERIODICALS

308 *American Journal of Occupational Therapy*. Rockville, MD: American Occupational Therapy Association. 12 pa. 1947–.

309 Unused.

310 *Australian Occupational Therapy Journal*. St Clair, NSW: Australian Association of Occupational Therapists. 4 pa. 1951–.

311 *British Journal of Occupational Therapy*. London: College of Occupational Therapists. 12 pa. 1974–.

312 *Canadian Journal of Occupational Therapy*. Toronto: Canadian Association of Occupational Therapists. 5 pa. 1933–.

313 *Contact*. London: RADAR. 4 pa. 1973–.

314 *Design for Special Needs*. London: Centre on Environment for the Handicapped. 3 pa. 1973–. (From 1990, *Access by Design*.)

315 *Occupational Therapy in Health Care*. New York: Haworth Press. 4 pa. 1984–.

316   *Occupational Therapy in Mental Health.* New York: Haworth Press. 4 pa. 1980–.

317   *Occupational Therapy Journal of Research.* Laurel, MD: American Occupational Therapy Foundation Inc. 6 pa. 1981–.

318   *OT Micronews.* 4 pa. 1984–. (Contact: Mrs C. V. MacCaul (Secretary), Senior Lecturer in Occupational Therapy, Christchurch College, North Holmes Road, Canterbury CT1 1QU, England.)

319   *OTSIGN Newsletter.* 2 pa. 1986–. (Contact: Hilary King, 19A Cowper Road, Wimbledon, London SW19 1AA.)

320   *Physical and Occupational Therapy in Geriatrics.* New York: Haworth Press. 4 pa. 1980–.

321   *Physical and Occupational Therapy in Pediatrics.* New York: Haworth Press. 4 pa. 1980–.

322   *PIP Newsletter.* 3 pa. 1982–. (From 1990, *NAPOT Newsletter.*) (Contact: Mary Jones (Membership secretary), Occupational Therapy Department, Chailey Heritage, North Chailey, Near Lewes, East Sussex BN8 4EF, England.)

323   *Radar Bulletin.* London: RADAR. 11 pa. 1972–.

CURRENT AWARENESS SOURCES, INDEXES AND ABSTRACTS

Applied Social Sciences Index and Abstracts, ASSIA [86].

324   *British Institute of Mental Handicap Current Awareness Service.* Kidderminster, Worcs.: BIMH. 26 pa.

Information Service Handbook (Disabled Living Foundation) [156].

Occupational Therapy Index [78].

RECAL [228].

Rehabilitation Bulletin (National Demonstration Centre, Pinderfields General Hospital) [92].

Rehabilitation Index [80].

325   *Information Directories.* Edinburgh: Disability Scotland. Irregular.

Terminal Care Index [81].

BIBLIOGRAPHIES

Most of the books mentioned below contain bibliographies. In addition:

326 *Bibliography on occupational therapy* (1981). WFOT. (Available from Mrs Barbara Posthuma, Department of Occupational Therapy, Health Sciences Centre, The University of Western Ontario, London, Ontario, Canada N6A 5C1.)

327 *Resource Papers*. London: Disabled Living Foundation.
These papers cover autobiographies, biographies and novels by or about disabled people; children; design and access; disabled people; elderly; independent living; lifting and handling the disabled person; mental handicap; multiple sclerosis; specific disabilities; stroke; wheelchairs; audio-visual material on disability. They give details of publications, audio-visual aids and specialist organizations.

328 **Ellis, R.** and **Margrain, S.** (1981). *Occupational therapy research: a bibliography with summaries*. Ulster: Ulster Polytechnic/COT.

329 *Bibliographies*. Edinburgh: Scottish Health Service Centre.
The library has several specialist bibliographies, some of which are relevant to occupational therapy. A list is available on application to the librarian. The library will also undertake literature searches. Library staff are in the process of developing a computerized database of books and journal articles held in the library.

330 **Williams, R.** (1986). *Information searching in health care: a workbook for occupational therapists and physiotherapists*. Hamilton, Ontario: McMaster University.

BOOKS

331 **Allen, C. K.** (1985). *Occupational therapy for psychiatric diseases: measurement and management of cognitive disabilities*. Boston: Little, Brown & Co. 408 pp.

332 **American Occupational Therapy Association** (1986). *Occupational therapy education: target 2000*. Rockville, MD: AOTA. 213 pp. (Proceedings of a colloquium held in Nashville, TN, 22–26 June 1986.)

333 **Andamo, E. M.** (1984). *Guide to program evaluation for physical therapy and occupational therapy services*. New York: Haworth Press. 151 pp.

334 **Axline, V.** (1989). *Play therapy*. Edinburgh: Churchill Livingstone. 350 pp.

335   Bair, J. and Gray, M., eds (1985). *The occupational therapy manager.* Rockville, MD: AOTA. 420 pp.

336   Barris, R., Kielhofner, G. and Watts, J. (1988). *Bodies of knowledge in psychosocial practice.* Thorofare, NJ: C. B. Slack. 172 pp.

337   Barris, R., Kielhofner, G. and Watts, J. (1988). *Occupational therapy in psychosocial practice.* Thorofare, NJ: C. B. Slack. 141 pp.

338   Bell, J. (1988). *Doing your research project.* Oxford: Oxford University Press. 145 pp.

339   Berry, H., Hamilton, E. and Goodwill, J., eds (1983). *Rheumatology and rehabilitation.* London: Croom Helm. 266 pp.

340   De Gilio, S., Bowden, R. and Burrows, H. (1989). *The management manual.* Bicester: Winslow Press. 112 pp.

341   Briggs, A. and Agrin, A. eds (1985). *Crossroads: a reader for psychosocial occupational therapy.* Rockville, MD: AOTA. 215 pp.

342   Bruce, M. A. and Borg, B. (1987). *Frames of reference in psychosocial occupational therapy.* Thorofare, NJ: C. B. Slack. 409 pp.

343   Bumphrey, E., ed. (1987). *Occupational therapy in the community.* Cambridge: Woodhead-Faulkner. 270 pp.

344   Burnard, P. (1989). *Counselling skills for health professionals.* London: Chapman & Hall. 201 pp.

345   Clarke, A. (1987). *Rehabilitation in rheumatology: the team approach.* London: Martin Dunitz. 320 pp.

346   College of Occupational Therapists (1984). *Resource book for community occupational therapists.* London: COT.

347   College of Occupational Therapists (1988). *Occupational therapists' reference book 1988.* Norwich: Parke Sutton/BAOT. 128 pp.

348   College of Occupational Therapists Research Committee (1985). *Research advice handbook for occupational therapists.* London: COT. 44 pp.
A new edition is in preparation.

349   **Crepeau, E.**, ed. (1986). *Activity programming for the elderly*. Boston: Little, Brown & Co. 164 pp.

350   **Cromwell, F.**, ed. (1984). *Occupational therapy and the patient with pain*. New York: Haworth Press. 135 pp.

351   **Cromwell, F.**, ed. (1986). *Computer applications in occupational therapy*. New York: Haworth Press. 200 pp.

352   **Darnbrough, A.** and **Kinrade, D.** (1986). *Directory of aids for disabled and elderly people*. Cambridge: Woodhead-Faulkner. 162 pp.

353   **DeLisa, J.**, ed. (1988). *Rehabilitation medicine: principles and practice*. Philadelphia: J. B. Lippincott. 903 pp.

354   **Denton, P.** (1987). *Psychiatric occupational therapy: a workbook of practical skills*. Boston: Little, Brown & Co. 192 pp.

355   **Eggers, O.** (1983). *Occupational therapy in the treatment of adult hemiplegia*. London: Heinemann. 150 pp.

356   **Ellis, R.**, ed. (1988). *Professional competence and quality assurance in the caring professions*. London: Croom Helm. 315 pp.

357   **Finlay, L.** (1988). *Occupational therapy practice in psychiatry*. London: Croom Helm. 162 pp.

358   **Fransella, F.** (1982). *Psychology for occupational therapists*. London: Macmillan. 368 pp.

359   **Fussey, I.** and **Giles, G. M.**, eds (1988). *Rehabilitation of the severely brain-injured adult*. London: Croom Helm. 233 pp.

360   **Goodgold, J.**, ed. (1988). *Rehabilitation medicine*. London: C. V. Mosby.

361   **Goodwill, C. J.** and **Chamberlain, M. A.**, eds (1988). *Rehabilitation of the physically disabled adult*. London: Croom Helm. 881 pp.

362   **Granger, C. V.**, **Seltzer, G. B.** and **Fishbein, C. F.** (1987). *Primary care of the functionally disabled: assessment and management*. Philadelphia: J. B. Lippincott. 417 pp.

363   **Harpin, P.** (1983). *With a little help*. London: Muscular Dystrophy Group. 8 volumes.

364   Helm, M. (1987). *Occupational therapy with the elderly*. Edinburgh: Churchill Livingstone. 271 pp.

365   Hemphill, B.T., ed. (1982). *The evaluative process in psychiatric occupational therapy*. Thorofare, NJ: C. B. Slack. 401 pp.

366   Hogg, J. and **Raynes, N.**, eds (1987). *Assessment in mental handicap: a guide to assessment, practices, tests and checklists*. London: Croom Helm. 289 pp.

367   Holden, U. P. (1984). *Thinking it through*. Bicester: Winslow Press. 46 pp.

368   Holden, U. P. and **Woods, R.T.** (1988). *Reality orientation: psychological approaches to the confused elderly*. 2nd ed. Edinburgh: Churchill Livingstone. 341 pp.

369   Hopkins, H. L. and **Smith, H. D.**, eds (1988). *Willard and Spackman's Occupational therapy*. 7th ed. Philadelphia: J. B. Lippincott. 863 pp.

370   Howe, M. C. and **Schwartzberg, S. L.** (1986). *A functional approach to group work in occupational therapy*. Philadelphia: J. B. Lippincott. 255 pp.

371   Hume, C. and **Pullen, I.** (1986). *Rehabilitation in psychiatry*. Edinburgh: Churchill Livingstone. 230 pp.

372   Isaac, D. (1989). *Community occupational therapy with mentally handicapped people*. London: Chapman & Hall.

373   Jacques, A. (1988). *Understanding dementia*. Edinburgh: Churchill Livingstone. 327 pp.

374   Jay, P. (1984). *Coping with disability*. London: Disabled Living Foundation. 208 pp.

375   Jennings, S. (1978). *Remedial drama*. London: Pitman. 144 pp.

376   Johnstone, M. (1987). *Home care for the stroke patient*. 2nd ed. Edinburgh: Churchill Livingstone. 218 pp.

377   Johnstone, M. (1987). *Restoration of motor function in the stroke patient*. 3rd ed. Edinburgh: Churchill Livingstone. 240 pp.

378   Johnstone, M. (1987). *The stroke patient: a team approach*. 3rd ed. Edinburgh: Churchill Livingstone. 114 pp.

379   Kielhofner, G. (1983). *Health through occupation.* Philadelphia, PA: F. A. Davis. 316 pp.

380   Kielhofner, G. (1985). *A model of human occupation.* Baltimore: Williams & Wilkins. 511 pp.

381   Knickerbocker, B. M. (1980). *A holistic approach to the treatment of learning disorders.* Thorofare, NJ: C. B. Slack. 387 pp.

382   Landgarten, H. B. (1981). *Clinical art therapy.* New York: Brunner/Mazel. 390 pp.

383   Latto, S. (1986). *Use of microcomputers in occupational therapy.* Liverpool: Liverpool Institute of Higher Education. 4 volumes.

384   Liebmann, M. (1986). *Art therapy for groups.* London: Croom Helm. 226 pp.

385   McCarthy, G. T. (1984). *The physically handicapped child: an interdisciplinary approach to management.* London: Faber & Faber. 375 pp.

386   Melvin, J. L. (1982). *Rheumatic disease: occupational therapy and rehabilitation.* 2nd ed. Philadelphia, PA: F. A. Davis. 428 pp.

387   Mills, D. and **Fraser C.** (1988). *Therapeutic activities for the upper limb.* Bicester: Winslow Press. 160 pp.

388   Mosey, A. C. (1970). *Three frames of reference for mental health.* Thorofare, NJ: C. B. Slack. 241 pp.

389   Mosey, A. C. (1973). *Activities therapy.* New York: Raven Press. 195 pp.

390   Mosey, A. C. (1981). *Occupational therapy: configuration of a profession.* New York: Raven Press. 173 pp.

391   Mosey, A. C. (1986). *Psychosocial components of occupational therapy.* New York: Raven Press. 606 pp.

392   O'Sullivan, S. and **Schmitz, T.** (1988). *Physical rehabilitation: assessment and treatment.* 2nd ed. Philadelphia, PA: F. A. Davis.

393   Ottenbacher, K. J. (1986). *Evaluating clinical change: strategies for occupational and physical therapists.* Baltimore, MD: Williams & Wilkins. 243 pp.

394 Unused.

395 **Peck, C.** and **Chia, S. H.** (1987). *Living skills for mentally handicapped people.* London: Croom Helm. 221 pp.

396 **Pedretti, L. W.** and **Zoltan, B.** (1990). *Occupational therapy: practice skills for physical dysfunction.* 3rd ed. St Louis, MO: C. V. Mosby. 690 pp.

397 **Penso, D.** (1987). *Occupational therapy for children with disabilities.* London: Croom Helm. 181 pp.

398 **Priestley, P.** and **McGuire, J.** (1983). *Learning to help: basic skills exercises.* London: Tavistock. 160 pp.

399 **Priestley, P.** *et al.* (1978). *Social skills and personal problem solving: a handbook of methods.* London: Tavistock. 203 pp.

400 **Reed, K.** (1984). *Models of practice in occupational therapy.* Baltimore, MD: Williams & Wilkins. 548 pp.

401 **Reed, K.** and **Sanderson, S. R.** (1980). *Concepts of occupational therapy.* Baltimore, MD: Williams & Wilkins. 297 pp.

402 **Remocker, A. J.** and **Storch, E. T.** (1987). *Action speaks louder: a handbook of non-verbal group techniques.* 4th ed. Edinburgh: Churchill Livingstone. 194 pp.

403 **Ridgway, L.** and **McKears, S.** (1985). *Computer help for disabled people.* London: Souvenir Press. 190 pp.

404 **Salter, M. I.** (1987). *Hand injuries: a therapeutic approach.* Edinburgh: Churchill Livingstone. 205 pp.

405 **Sandhu, J.** and **Richardson, S.** (1989). *The concerned technology 1989.* Newcastle upon Tyne: Handicapped Persons Research Unit. 228 pp.

406 **Saunders, P.** (1984). *Micros for handicapped users.* Whitby, N. Yorks.: Helena Press. 187 pp.

407 **Schwartz, R. K.** (1985). *Therapy as learning.* Dubuque, IA: Kendal Hunt. 139 pp.

408 **Scott, D.** and **Katz, N.**, eds (1988). *Occupational therapy in mental health: principles in practice.* London: Taylor & Francis. 222 pp.

409   Shanley, E., ed. (1986). *Mental handicap: a handbook of care*. Edinburgh: Churchill Livingstone. 336 pp.

410   Squires, A. J., ed. (1988). *Rehabilitation of the older patient*. London: Croom Helm. 279 pp.

411   Trombly, C. A., ed. (1989). *Occupational therapy for physical dysfunction*. 3rd ed. Baltimore, MD: Williams & Wilkins. 629 pp.

412   Turner, A., ed. (1987). *The practice of occupational therapy*. 2nd ed. Edinburgh: Churchill Livingstone. 593 pp.

413   Warren, B., ed. (1984). *Using the creative arts in therapy*. London: Croom Helm. 173 pp.

414   Weyers, J. (1986). *Wheelchairs and their use – a guide to choosing a wheelchair*. London: RADAR. 424 pp.

415   Wilcock, A. A. (1986). *Occupational therapy approaches to stroke*. Edinburgh: Churchill Livingstone. 235 pp.

416   Willson, M. (1987). *Occupational therapy in long-term psychiatry*. 2nd ed. Edinburgh: Churchill Livingstone. 222 pp.

417   Willson, M. (1988). *Occupational therapy in short-term psychiatry*. 2nd ed. Edinburgh: Churchill Livingstone. 320 pp.

418   Wing, J. and **Morris, B.** (1981). *Handbook of psychiatric rehabilitation practice*. Oxford: Oxford University Press. 188 pp.

419   World Federation of Occupational Therapists. Proceedings of international congresses:

First (1954). *Proceedings of first international congress*. Edinburgh.

Second (1958). *Occupational therapy as a link in rehabilitation*. Copenhagen.

Third (1962). *Cultural patterns affecting rehabilitation*. Philadelphia, PA.

Fourth (1966). *Through youth to age*. London.

Fifth (1970). *Occupational therapy today – tomorrow*. Munich.

Sixth (1974). *Health care in the seventies*. Vancouver, BC.

Seventh (1978). *Occupational therapy in a changing world*. Jerusalem.

Eighth (1982). *Occupational therapy and rehabilitation: Help for the handicapped.* Hamburg.

Ninth (1986). Congress cancelled.

(Information on the above proceedings can be obtained from the Honorary Secretary of the World Federation of Occupational Therapists – see Part III [1016].)

DATABASES

420   *BARD: British Database on Research into Aids for the Disabled*
Based at the Handicapped Persons Research Unit at Newcastle upon Tyne Polytechnic, BARD contains over 1000 records since 1984, on British design and development works, prototypes, research projects, surveys, evaluations. Information is available as printed lists.

421   *BARDSOFT*
Also based at the Handicapped Persons Research Unit at Newcastle upon Tyne Polytechnic, this database contains about 2000 software programs (for over 40 types of microcomputer) for people with special needs; their descriptor headings are: assessment, cognition, employment, language, numeracy, perception/ motor, recreation, teaching, training/therapy, general.

422   *RECAL Offline*
Over 14 000 bibliographic records from over 100 periodicals taken at the National Centre for Training and Education in Prosthetics and Orthotics at the University of Strathclyde; available for use on IBM PC/XT or AT computers.

423   *SCD-DATA*
Available from Disability Scotland in Edinburgh. Based on the Disabled Living Foundation's aids and equipment database with the addition of information on holidays, voluntary organizations and Scottish suppliers. Subscribers have access using basic desk-top or portable computers.

424   *Help for Health Information Service*
Run and funded by the Wessex Regional Health Authority, this is a microcomputer based system with a database containing details of over 3000 mainly English self-help organizations, more than 2000 leaflets and pamphlets and at least 800 publications.

425   *Health Search Scotland*
Health information and resources service from the Scottish Health Education Group, which aims to provide comprehensive, regularly updated information on

national and local self-help and voluntary groups concerned with health throughout Scotland.

426   DLF-DATA
The Disabled Living Foundation's computerized database of products, technical aids and associated advice notes. An advanced system with fast accurate recall of information by almost any search term.

REPORTS

427   Beardshaw, V. (1988). *Last on the list: community services for people with physical disabilities*. London: King's Fund.

428   British Association of Occupational Therapists (1981). *The way ahead: report of the Working Party*. London: BAOT.

429   College of Occupational Therapists (1983). *The case for a degree in occupational therapy*. Paper by the Education Board and approved by Council. London: COT.

430   College of Occupational Therapists (1981). *Diploma course 1981: training in occupational therapy*. London: COT.

431   Council for Professions Supplementary to Medicine (1973). *Report of the Remedial Professions Committee*. London: CPSM. Burt Report.

432   Department of Health. *Disability Equipment Assessment Programmes*. London: DHSS. Obtainable from DHSS Health Publications Unit, Heywood, Lancs.

433   Department of Health and Social Security (1972). *Rehabilitation*. Report of a Sub-Committee of the Standing Medical Advisory Committee, chairman, Sir R. E. Tunbridge. London: HMSO. 187 pp.

434   Department of Health and Social Security (1973). *The remedial professions*. Report by a Working Party, chairman E. L. McMillan. London: HMSO. 24 pp.

435   Department of Health and Social Security (1975). *Report of the Committee of Inquiry into the pay and related conditions of service of the professions supplementary to medicine and speech therapists*, chairman the Earl of Halsbury. London: HMSO.

436   Department of Health and Social Security (1986). *Clinical and managerial information systems for physiotherapy and occupational therapy*. London: HMSO.

437 **Department of Health and Social Security** (1988). *Community care: agenda for action*. A report to the Secretary of State for Social Sciences, by Sir R. Griffiths. London: HMSO.

438 **Department of Health and Social Security** (1988). *Equipment and services for disabled people*. London: HMSO. Leaflet HB6.

439 **Department of Health and Social Security** (1988). *Resourcing the National Health Service: short-term issues*. First reports of the Social Services Committee. London: HMSO. 3 volumes.

439a **Independent Commission into Occupational Therapy** (1989). *Occupational therapy: an emerging profession in health care*, chairman L. Blom-Cooper. London: Duckworth.

440 **Independent Development Council for People with Mental Handicap** (1988). *Frameworks for change*. London: King's Fund.

441 **International Round Table for The Advancement of Counselling** (1988). *Counselling disabled people and their families*. Penarth: IRTAC.

442 **Johnson, H.** and **Paterson, C. F.** (1975). *Training for the remedial professions*. London: King's Fund.

443 **National Association of Health Authorities** (1986). *Recruitment and retention of staff in the professions supplementary to medicine*. Birmingham: NAHA.

444 **National Audit Office** (1986). *National Health Service: control over professional and technical manpower*. London: HMSO.

445 **National Audit Office** (1987). *Making a reality of community care*. London: HMSO.

446 **Tracey, R. T.** (1976–81). *Integrating the disabled*. Report of a Working Party of the National Fund for Research into Crippling Diseases, chairman the Earl of Snowdon. London: NFRCD. 3 volumes.

447 **Occupational Therapists' Board** (1972). *Future education and training of occupational therapists*. London: CPSM.

448 **Stewart, A.** (1979). *Study of occupational therapy teaching resources in the United Kingdom*. Report to the Occupational Therapists' Board. London: CPSM.

449 **Harris, A.** (1971). *Handicapped and impaired in Great Britain*. Report to the Office of Population Censuses and Surveys. London: HMSO.

450   Review Body for Nursing Staff, Midwives, Health Visitors and Professions Allied to Medicine (1984). *Second report on the professions allied to medicine* . . ., chairman Sir J. H. Greenborough. London: HMSO. 32 pp.

450a   Review Body for Nursing Staff, Midwives, Health Visitors and Professions Allied to Medicine (1988). *Fifth report on the professions allied to medicine* . . ., chairman Sir J. Cleminson. Cmnd 361. London: HMSO.

451   Royal College of Physicians (1986). Physical disability in 1986 and beyond. *Journal of the Royal College of Physicians*, **20**, 160–94.

452   Scottish Association of Occupational Therapy (1971). *Review of educational policy*. Report of a Working Party and recommendations to the Board of Studies. Edinburgh: SAOT. Shaw Report.

453   Scottish Health Service Planning Council (1980). *Occupational therapy staffing survey in Scotland 1980*, survey co-ordinator C. F. Paterson. Edinburgh: Scottish Health Service Centre.

454   Scottish Home and Health Department. *Help for handicapped people in Scotland*. Edinburgh: HMSO. Leaflet HB1(S).

455   Scottish Home and Health Department (1972). *Medical rehabilitation: the pattern for the future*. Report of a Sub-Committee of the Standing Medical Advisory Committee, chairman A. Mair. Edinburgh: HMSO.

456   Scottish Home and Health Department (1984). *The role of the paramedical professions*. A report by the National Paramedical (Therapeutic) Consultative Committee. Edinburgh: HMSO.

457   Scottish Home and Health Department (1987). *Five health professions: guidance to health boards*. Edinburgh: HMSO.

458   Scottish Home and Health Department (1988). *A survey of aids and equipment for disabled people in Scotland*. A report prepared by the Committee for Research on Equipment for the Disabled. Edinburgh: HMSO.

459   World Federation of Occupational Therapists (1985). *Recommended minimum standards for the education of occupational therapists*. London, Ontario: WFOT.

4 Physiotherapy
Graham Walton

JOURNALS

460 *Physiotherapy*. London: Chartered Society of Physiotherapy. 12 pa. 1915–. etc

461 *Nederlands Tijdschrift voor Fysiotherapie*. Amersfoort: Nederlands Genootschap voor Fysiotherapie. 6 pa. 1890–.

462 *American Journal of Physical Medicine and Rehabilitation*. Baltimore, MD: Williams & Wilkins. 6 pa. 1921–.

463 *Archives of Physical Medicine and Rehabilitation*. Chicago, IL: American Congress of Rehabilitation. 12 pa. 1921–.

464 *Australian Journal of Physiotherapy*. North Fitzroy: Australian Physiotherapy Association. 12 pa. 1954–.

465 *Physical Therapy*. Fairfax, VA: American Physical Therapy Association. 12 pa. 1921–.

466 *Physiotherapie*. Lubeck, FRG: Verlag Otto Haase. 12 pa.

467 *Physiotherapy Canada*. Toronto: Canadian Physiotherapy Association. 6 pa. 1923–.

468 *South African Journal of Physiotherapy*. Parklands: Medical Association of South Africa on behalf of the South African Society of Physiotherapy. 12 pa. 1944–.

469 *Journal of Orthopaedic and Sports Physical Therapy*. Baltimore, MD: Orthopaedic and Sports Physical Therapy Section of the American Physical Therapy Association. 6 pa. 1979–.

470 *Clinical Management in Physical Therapy*. Alexandria, VA: American Physical Therapy Association. 6 pa. 1980–.

471 *Physiotherapy Practice*. Edinburgh: Churchill Livingstone. 4 pa. 1984–.

472 *Physical Therapy in Health Care*. New York: Hawarth Press. 4 pa. 1986–.

CURRENT AWARENESS SOURCES

473 *Current Contents: Clinical Medicine*. Philadelphia, PA: Institute for Scientific Information. 52 pa. 1973–.

474 *Current Contents: Life Sciences*. Philadelphia, PA: Institute for Scientific Information. 52 pa. 1958–.

475 *Current Contents: Social and Behavioral Sciences*. Philadelphia, PA: Institute for Scientific Information. 52 pa. 1969–.

Physiotherapy Index [79].

Rehabilitation Index [80].

INDEXES AND ABSTRACTS

Applied Social Sciences Index and Abstracts, ASSIA [86].

Cumulative Index to Nursing and Allied Health Literature, CINAHL [69].

476 *Excerpta Medica: Rehabilitation and Physical Medicine*. Amsterdam: Elsevier Science Publishers. 10 pa. 1958–.

Health Service Abstracts [71].

Hospital Literature Index [88].

Index Medicus [58].

REFERENCE BOOKS

477 *Chartered physiotherapists' source book.* (1987). 2nd ed. Norwich: Parke Sutton Publishing. 225 pp.

478 Gibson, A., ed. (1988). *Physiotherapy in the community.* Cambridge: Woodhead-Faulkner. 294 pp.

479 National Association of Health Authorities, NAHA (1987). *NHS handbook.* 3rd ed. London: Macmillan. 203 pp.

480 *Physiotherapists' Register 1987/88* (1987). London: Council for Professions Supplementary to Medicine. 447 pp.

481 Fry, J. *et al.* (1985). *Disease data book.* Lancaster: MTP Press. 405 pp.

482 *Chartered Society of Physiotherapy, Research and evaluation register.* London: Chartered Society of Physiotherapy. Annual. 1987–.

Bibliographies

483 Lloyd, H. A. and **Fraser, M. D. E.** (1977). *The information needs of physiotherapists in the Atlantic provinces with suggested physiotherapy working collections for small hospitals.* Halifax, Nova Scotia: Dalhousie University Libraries/ Dalhousie University School of Library Service. 39 pp.

484 Fraser, M. D. E. and **Lloyd, H.A.** (1981). *Information needs of physiotherapists, with a guide to physiotherapy collections for community general hospitals.* 2nd ed. Halifax, Nova Scotia: Dalhousie University School of Library Service. 72 pp.

485 Patrias, K., compiler (1988). *Physical fitness and sports medicine: June 1988: 1406 selected citations.* Bethesda, MD: National Library of Medicine. 62 pp.

486 *British National Bibliography.* London: British Library Bibliographical Services Division. 52 pa. 1950–.

487 *British Medicine.* Oxford: Pergamon Press. 12 pa. 1972–.

BOOKS

488 Downie, P.A., ed. (1987). *Cash's Textbook of chest, heart and vascular disorders for physiotherapists.* 4th ed. London: Faber & Faber. 704 pp.

489   Downie, P.A., ed. (1984). *Cash's Textbook of general medical and surgical conditions for physiotherapists*. London: Faber & Faber. 462 pp.

490   Downie, P.A., ed. (1986). *Cash's Textbook of neurology for physiotherapists*. 4th ed. London: Faber and Faber. 653 pp.

491   Downie, P.A., ed. (1984). *Cash's Textbook of orthopaedics and rheumatology for physiotherapists*. London: Faber & Faber. 638 pp.

492   French, M. (1987). *A career in physiotherapy*. London: Batsford. 112 pp.

493   Carr, J. H. and **Shepherd, R.B.**, (1987). *Foundations for physical therapy in stroke rehabilitation*. London: Heinemann. 186 pp.

494   Downer, A. H. (1978). *Physical therapy procedures*. 3rd ed. Springfield, IL: Charles C. Thomas. 306 pp.

495   Arnould-Taylor, W. E. (1982). *The principles and practice of physical therapy*. 2nd ed. Cheltenham: Stanley Thornes (Publishers). 189 pp.

496   Lee, J., ed. (1988). *Aids to physiotherapy*. 2nd ed. Edinburgh: Churchill Livingstone. 204 pp.

497   Buchele, M. and **Wynn-Williams, S.** (1987). *Successful private practice; guide to effective medical practice management*. Edinburgh: Churchill Livingstone. 238 pp.

498   Moffat, D. B. (1986). *Anatomy and physiology for physiotherapists*. 2nd ed. London: Blackwell Scientific Press. 320 pp.

499   Williams, P. L. and **Warwick, R.**, eds (1980). *Gray's Anatomy*. 36th ed. Edinburgh: Churchill Livingstone. 1578 pp.

500   Parry, A. (1985). *Physiotherapy assessment: an introduction*. 2nd ed. London: Croom Helm. 160 pp.

501   Cole, J. H. (1988). *Muscles in action: an approach to manual muscle testing*. Edinburgh: Churchill Livingstone. 168 pp.

502   Coates, H. and **King, A.** (1982). *The patient assessment: a handbook for therapists*. Edinburgh: Churchill Livingstone. 144 pp.

503   Rothstein, J. M., ed. (1985). *Measurement in physical therapy*. Edinburgh: Churchill Livingstone. 311 pp. (Clinics in Physical Therapy series.)

504   **Payton, O. D.**, ed. (1986). *Interpersonal relationships with patients: psychological aspects of clinical practice.* Edinburgh: Churchill Livingstone. 161 pp. (Clinics in Physical Therapy series.)

505   **Bourne, D.** (1981). *Under the doctor: studies in the psychological problems of physiotherapists, patients and doctors.* Amersham, Bucks.: Avebury Publishing Company. 211 pp.

506   **Dunkin, N.** (1981). *Psychology for physiotherapists.* Basingstoke: Macmillan. 401 pp.

507   **Hare, M.** (1986). *Physiotherapy in psychiatry.* London: Heinemann. 195 pp.

Electrotherapy, Exercise and Manipulation

508   **Forster, A.** and **Palastanga, N.** (1985). *Clayton's Electrotherapy: theory and practice.* 9th ed. London: Baillière Tindall. 232 pp.

509   **Kahn, J.** (1987). *Principles and practice of electrotherapy.* Edinburgh: Churchill Livingstone. 200 pp.

510   **Wolf, S. L.**, ed. (1981). *Electrotherapy.* Edinburgh: Churchill Livingstone. 204 pp. (Clinics in Physical Therapy series.)

511   **Nikolova, L.** (1987). *Treatment with interferential currrent.* Edinburgh: Churchill Livingstone. 190 pp.

512   **Sjolund, B.** and **Eriksson, M.** (1985). *Relief of pain by TENS: transcutaneous electrical nerve stimulation.* Chichester: John Wiley. 116 pp.

513   **Wells, P. E.** *et al.* (1988). *Pain: management and control in physiotherapy.* London: Heinemann. 316 pp.

514   **Colson, J. H. C.** and **Collison, F. W.** (1983). *Progressive exercise therapy in rehabilitation and physical education.* 4th ed. Bristol: John Wright. 284 pp.

515   **Sullivan, P. E.** *et al.* (1982). *An integrated approach to therapeutic exercise.* Reston, VA: Reston Publishing Company. 362 pp.

516   **Wale, J. O.**, ed. (1968). *Tidy's Massage and remedial exercises.* 11th ed. Bristol: John Wright. 510 pp.

517   **Hollis, M.** (1987). *Massage for therapists.* Oxford: Blackwell Scientific Publications. 115 pp.

518   Bourdillon, J. F. and **Day, E. A.** (1987). *Spinal manipulation*. 4th ed. London: Heinemann. 250 pp.

519   Glasgow, E. F., ed. (1985). *Aspects of manipulative therapy*. 2nd ed. Melbourne: Churchill Livingstone. 194 pp.

520   Maitland, G. D. (1986). *Vertebral manipulation*. 5th ed. London: Butterworths. 390 pp.

521   Pelosi, T. and **Gleeson, M.** (1987). *Illustrated transfer techniques for disabled people*. Melbourne: Churchill Livingstone. 180 pp.

Normal Movement

522   Galley, P. M. and **Forster, A. L.** (1987). *Human movement: an introductory text for physiotherapy students*. 2nd ed. Edinburgh: Churchill Livingstone. 262 pp.

523   Gowtizke, B. A. and **Milner, M.** (1988). *Understanding the scientific basis of human movement*. 3rd ed. Baltimore, MD: Williams & Wilkins. 432 pp.

524   Carr, J. H. (1987). *Movement science: foundations for physical therapy in rehabilitation*. London: Heinemann.

Life Continuum

525   McKenna, J., ed. (1987). *Obstetrics and gynaecology*. Edinburgh: Churchill Livingstone. 191 pp. (International Perspectives in Physical Therapy series.)

526   Scrutton, D. and **Gilbertson, M.** (1975). *Physiotherapy in paediatric practice*. London: Butterworths. 205 pp.

527   Shepherd, R. B. (1980). *Physiotherapy in paediatrics*. 2nd ed. London: Heinemann. 524 pp.

528   Campion, M. R. (1985). *Hydrotherapy in paediatrics*. London: Heinemann. 265 pp.

529   Hawker, M. (1985). *The older patient and the role of the physiotherapist*. 2nd ed. London: Faber & Faber. 167 pp.

530   Jackson, O. (1983). *Physical therapy of the geriatric patient*. Edinburgh: Churchill Livingstone. 239 pp. (Clinics in Physical Therapy series.)

531   Wagstaff, P. and **Coakley, D.** (1988). *Physiotherapy and the elderly patient*. London: Croom Helm. 224 pp.

Neurology

532   **Carr, J. H.** and **Shepherd, R. B.** (1980). *Physiotherapy in disorders of the brain*. London: Heinemann. 416 pp.

533   **Bethlem, J.** and **Knobbout, C. E.** (1987). *Neuromuscular diseases*. Oxford: Oxford University Press. 158 pp.

534–536   Unused.

537   **Banks, M. A.**, ed. (1986). *Stroke*. Edinburgh: Churchill Livingstone. 225 pp. (International Perspectives in Physical Therapy series.)

538   **Carr, J. H.** and **Shepherd, R. B.** (1987). *A motor relearning programme for stroke*. 2nd ed. London: Heinemann. 208 pp.

Cardiopulmonary

539   **Gaskell, D. V.** (1980). *The Brompton Hospital Guide to chest physiotherapy*. 4th ed. London: Blackwell Scientific Press. 120 pp.

540   **Irwin, S.** and **Tecklin, J. S.**, eds (1985). *Cardiopulmonary physical therapy*. St Louis, MO: C. V. Mosby. 423 pp.

541   **Hall, K. K.**, ed. (1984). *Cardiac rehabilitation: exercise testing and prescription*. Lancaster: MTP Press. 452 pp.

542   **Frownfelter, D. L.** (1987). *Chest physical therapy and pulmonary rehabilitation: an interdisciplinary approach*. 2nd ed. Chicago, IL: Year Book Medical Publishers. 794 pp.

Orthopaedics

543   **Engstrom, B.** and **Van de Ven, C.** (1985). *Physiotherapy for amputees: the Roehampton approach*. Edinburgh: Churchill Livingstone. 289 pp.

544   **Mensch, G.** and **Ellis, P. M.** (1987). *Physical therapy management of lower extremity amputations*. London: Heinemann. 365 pp.

545   **Salter, M.** (1987). *Hand injuries: a therapeutic approach*. Edinburgh: Churchill Livingstone. 205 pp.

546   **Kuprian, W.**, ed. (1982). *Physical therapy for sports*. Philadelphia, PA: W. B. Saunders. 377 pp.

547   Gould, J. A. and **Davies, G. J.**, eds (1989). *Orthopaedic and sports physical therapy.* 2nd ed. St Louis, MO: C. V. Mosby. 700 pp.

548   Davies, P. M. (1985). *Steps to follow: a guide to the treatment of hemiplegia.* Berlin: Springer-Verlag. 300 pp.

549   Nixon, V. (1985). *Spinal cord injury: a guide to functional outcomes in physical therapy management.* Rockville, MD: Aspen. 228 pp.

550   Bromley, I. (1985). *Tetraplegia and paraplegia.* Edinburgh: Churchill Livingstone. 264 pp.

551   Hyde, S. A. (1980). *Physiotherapy in rheumatology.* Oxford: Blackwell Scientific Press. 100 pp.

552   Unused.

Research

553   Payton, O. D. (1988). *Research: the validation of clinical practice.* 2nd ed. Philadelphia, PA: F. A. Davis. 311 pp.

554   APTA (1983). *Research: an anthology.* Alexandria, VA: American Physical Therapy Association. 552 pp.

555   Currier, D. P. (1984). *Elements of research in physical therapy.* 2nd ed. Baltimore, MD: Williams & Wilkins. 341 pp.

REPORTS

556   Ministry of Health and Department of Health for Scotland (1951). Report of the Committees on Medical Auxiliaries: Sir V. Z. Cope, chairman. Cmnd 8188. London: HMSO. 25 pp.

557   Fordham, R. and **Hodkinson, C.** (no date). *A cost–benefit-analysis of open access to physiotherapy for GPs.* York: Centre for Health Economics, York University. 45 pp.

558   Glossop, E. S. and **Smith, D. S.** (1979). *Domiciliary physiotherapy: a research report.* Brent: Brent and Harrow Health Authority. 30 pp.

559   Partridge, C. J. (1984). *Community physiotherapy and direct access to physiotherapy services by general practitioners within the NHS.* London: King's College. 30 pp.

560   **Körner, E.**, chairman (1984). *Steering Group on Health Services Information: fourth report to the Secretary of State*. London: HMSO. 49 pp.

CONFERENCES

561   **South African Society of Physiotherapy** (1983). *National congress: papers.* 262 pp.

562   **Chartered Society of Physiotherapy** (1978). Annual Congress – selected lectures 1978. *Physiotherapy*, **64** (12), whole issue.

563   **Canadian Physiotherapy Association** (1983). 1983: at the crossroads. *Physiotherapy Canada*, **35** (3), 241–79.

564   **Netherlands Society of Physiotherapy** (1977). European physiotherapy: fact or fiction? Spring symposium of the Netherlands Society of Physiotherapy. *Nederlands Tijdschrift voor Fysiotherapie*, **87** (7/8), 191–263.

565   **Titchen, A.**, ed. (1987). *Health education and physiotherapy: a venture in collaboration*. London: Health Education Authority. 35 pp.

566   **Docker, M. F.** ed. (1982). *Physics in physiotherapy: proceedings of the Hospital Physicists' Association and Chartered Society of Physiotherapy joint meeting, 2nd March 1980*. London: Hospital Physicists' Association. 42 pp.

AUDIO-VISUAL MATERIALS

567   **Hayne, C. R.** (1983). *Safe handling and lifting in hospital. 1, Basic introduction*. Chelmsford: Graves Medical Audio Visual Library. Video, 23 minutes.

567a   **Hayne, C. R.** (1983). *Safe handling and lifting in hospital. 2, Aids to manual lifting*. Chelmsford: Graves Medical AudioVisual Library. Video, 15 minutes.

568   **Bryant, B.** and **Roden, A.** (1977). *Bobath approach to adult hemiplegia*. Chelmsford: Graves Medical AudioVisual Library. Tape–slide, 36 minutes.

569   **Lowndes, S.** (1977). *Physiotherapy for children with asthma*. Chelmsford: Graves Medical AudioVisual Library. Tape–slide, 20 minutes.

570   **BMA/BLITHE Film and Video Library** (1988). *Medical films and videos from the BMA/BLITHE Film and Video Library*. London: BMA/BLITHE Film and Video Library.

5 Dietetics

Cathy Hyland and Karen Hyland

ABSTRACTS

571 *Food Science and Technology Abstracts.* Slough: Commonwealth Agricultural Bureaux. 12 pa. 1969–.
Scientific aspects of food technology.

572 *Health Education Index.* London: B. Edsall. Annual. 1973–.
A classified list of resources for health education.

573 *Nutrition Abstracts and Reviews.* Slough: Commonwealth Agricultural Bureaux. 12 pa. 1931–.

574 *Nutrition Reviews.* New York, NY: Springer. 12 pa. 1942–.

PERIODICALS

Dietetics and Nutrition

575 **Bush, R.** (1988). An annotated bibliography of journals in nutrition. *Serials Review*, 4, 35–43.
A detailed examination of 35 core periodicals.

576 *American Journal of Clinical Nutrition.* Baltimore, MD: American Society of Clinical Nutrition. 12 pa. 1954–.
Original research on nutrition and dietetics.

576a   *British Dietetic Association Adviser*. Birmingham: BDA. 4 pa. 1981–. Free to members.

576b   *British Dietetic Association Newsletter*. Birmingham: BDA. 12 pa. 1970–. Free to members.

577   *British Journal of Nutrition*. Cambridge: Cambridge University Press for the Nutrition Society. 6 pa. 1947–.

578   *Care of the Elderly*. London: Newbourne Group. 6 pa. 1989–. Multidisciplinary; medical and paramedical review articles.

579   *European Journal of Clinical Nutrition*. Continuation of *Human Nutrition* [591], [592]. Basingstoke: Macmillan. 12 pa. 1987–. Original articles and reviews.

580   *Food Additives and Contaminants*. London: Taylor & Francis. 4 pa. 1984–. Scientific aspects.

581   *Food Books Review*. Orpington, Kent: Food Trade Press. 4 pa. 1973–.

582   *Food Magazine*. London: London Food Commission. 12 pa. 1979–.

583   *Food Manufacture*. London: Morgan-Grampian. 12 pa. 1927–. Food industry review.

584   *Food Microbiology*. London: Academic Press. 4 pa. 1984–.

585   *Food Policy*. Sevenoaks, Kent: Butterworths. 4 pa. 1975–.

586   *Food Policy Research Briefing Papers*. Bradford: University of Bradford. Irregular. 1985–.

587   *Food Processing*. Orpington, Kent: Technical Press Publishing. 12 pa. 1931–. Scientific aspects of food technology.

588   *Food Sciences and Nutrition*. Continuation of *Human Nutrition: Food Science and Nutrition* [593]. Basingstoke: Macmillan. 4 pa. 1988–. Original articles and reviews.

589   *Gastroenterology*. Amsterdam: Elsevier. 12 pa. Clinical and basic studies of the digestive tract and liver; research papers and case reports.

590   *Gut*. London: British Medical Association. 12 pa. 1960–.
Journal of the British Society of Gastroenterology; nutrition and medical research.

591   *Human Nutrition: Applied Nutrition*. Continued as *European Journal of Clinical Nutrition* [579]. London: John Libbey for the BDA. 1947–1987.
Original articles and reviews on applied nutrition.

592   *Human Nutrition: Clinical Nutrition*. Continued as *European Journal of Clinical Nutrition* [579]. London: John Libbey for the BDA. 1947–1987.
Original articles and reviews relating to metabolic and nutrition responses and requirements, particularly in the care of the critically ill.

593   *Human Nutrition: Food Science and Nutrition*. Continued as *Food Science and Nutrition* [588].

594   *International Journal of Eating Disorders*. New York, NY: John Wiley. 6 pa. 1981–.

595   *International Journal of Obesity*. Basingstoke: Macmillan. 6 pa. 1976–. (From 1990, 12 pa.)
Original articles and research on obesity.

596   *Journal of Human Nutrition and Dietetics*. Oxford: Blackwell Scientific for the BDA. 4 pa. 1987–.
Original papers on human nutrition in health and disease, applied nutrition and dietetics.

597   *Journal of Micronutrient Analysis*. Amsterdam: Elsevier. 4 pa. 1985–.
Scientific aspects.

598   *Journal of Nutrition, Growth and Cancer*. London: John Libbey. 4 pa. 1983–.
Reviews on experimental and clinical cancer research and nutrition.

599   *Journal of the American Dietetic Association*. Chicago, IL: American Dietetic Association. 12 pa. 1925–.

600   *Journal of the Canadian Dietetic Association*. Toronto: Canadian Dietetic Association. 4 pa. 1967–.

601   *Nutrition Bulletin*. London: British Nutrition Foundation. 3 pa.
Original articles.

602   *Nutrition and Food Science* (continuation of *Review of Nutrition and Food Science*). London: Forbes Publications. 6 pa. 1965–.
On food, nutrition and nutrition education.

603   *Nutrition Research*. Oxford: Pergamon. 12 pa. 1981–.
Life sciences and medical aspects.

604   *Proceedings of the Nutrition Society*. Cambridge: Cambridge University Press.
3 pa. 1941–.
Nutrition reports, transactions and proceedings.

605   *Progress in Food and Nutrition Science*. Oxford: Pergamon. 4 pa. 1975–.
Life sciences and medical aspects.

606   *Progress in Lipid Research*. Oxford: Pergamon. 4 pa. 1952–.
Life science and medical aspects of lipid research; formerly *Progress in the Chemistry of Fats and Other Lipids*.

607   *What Diet and Lifestyle*. London: AIM Publications. 12 pa. 1984–.
Material collected together as *Diet and lifestyle book*.

Diabetes

608   *Diabetes: Journal of the American Diabetes Association*. Alexandria, VA: ADA.
12 pa.
Diabetes research.

609   *Diabetes Newsline*. London: British Diabetic Association. 3 pa.
For paramedical staff interested in diabetes.

610   *Diabetes Research and Clinical Practice*. Amsterdam: Elsevier. 6 pa.
Original international research articles and reviews, covering epidemiology, experimental biology, nutrition and clinical practice in diabetes.

611   *Diabetic Life*. London: National Diabetes Foundation. 4 pa. 1983–.

612   *Diabetic Medicine*. New York, NY: John Wiley. 12 pa. 1984–.
Diabetes research and multidisciplinary diabetes education.

613   *Diabetologia*. Heidelberg: Springer-Verlag. 12 pa.
Scientific aspects of clinical and experimental work on all aspects of diabetes research.

BOOKS

For ease of reference and use, particularly for departmental heads and specialist dietitians, the books are subdivided under main subject headings. The books recommended by training colleges and dietitians working in specialist fields are marked *; these titles are recommended for nutrition and dietetic department collections.

General Dietetics

*614   Alpers, D., Clouse, R. and **Stenson, W.** (1986). *Manual of nutritional therapeutics*. 4th ed. Boston, MA: Little, Brown. 457 pp.

615   Bennion, M. (1979). *Clinical nutrition*. London: Harper and Row. 564 pp.

616   Bodinsky, L. H. (1987). *Nurses' guide to diet therapy*. New York: John Wiley. 512 pp.

*617   Davidson, S. *et al.* (1986). *Human nutrition and dietetics*. 8th ed. Edinburgh: Churchill Livingstone. 666 pp.
An excellent reference book, with sections on physiology, nutritional disorders, food public health, diet and other disorders.

*618   Department of Health and Social Security (1988). *Catering for health: the recipe file*. London: HMSO. 292 pp.
A collection of 250 'healthy eating' recipes reflecting current nutritional recommendations.

*619   Department of Health and Social Security (1986). *Health service catering nutrition and modified diets*. 3rd ed. London: DHSS. 74 pp.
Intended primarily for use in hospital catering departments and by hospital nursing staff, it is also a useful reference in schools of nursing and colleges. The information is practical and considers the nutritional needs of *all* patients.

620   Department of Health (1989). *Chilled and frozen: guidelines on cook chill and cook freeze catering systems*. London: HMSO. 31 pp.
The guidelines combine and update the existing DHSS guidance on pre-cooked chilled and pre-cooked frozen foods and apply only to catering operations. They do not give guidance on chilled foods produced under special conditions using processes and packaging designed to provide an expected shelf-life of more than five days.

*621   Dickerson, J. and **Lee, H.** (1988). *Nutrition in the clinical management of disease*. 2nd ed. Oxford: Blackwell Scientific. 409 pp.
A system-by-system guide to nutrition in the prevention, treatment and control of diseases, integrating the pathophysiology and treatment of disease. The team approach to patient care is emphasized; additional literature is listed. Useful for those undertaking research on clinical nutrition.

*622   **Goode, A. W., Howard, J. P.** and **Woods, S.** (1985). *Clinical nutrition and dietetics for nurses*. Sevenoaks, Kent: Hodder & Stoughton. 214 pp.
Comprehensively explores nutrition and dietetics with reference to feeding patients in hospital, and major types of diet and treatment. The information is presented in an easy to understand and straightforward manner, particularly suitable for medical students, paramedical, nursing and catering staff.

623   **Harrison, R. J.** (1985). *Textbook of medicine*. 3rd ed. Sevenoaks, Kent: Hodder & Stoughton. 489 pp.
A highly readable, concise and clear textbook to help the reader understand and assimilate everyday medicine.

624   **Huskisson, J. M.** (1981). *Nutrition and dietetics in health and disease*. London: Baillière Tindall. 318 pp.
In two parts: part 1 considers the application of principles of nutrition in the diets of healthy people at all stages of life; part 2 deals with the physiology, dietetic theory and diets used in the treatment of various disease conditions.

625   **Hutchinson, E.** (1961). *A history of the British Dietetic Association, 1936–1961*. London: Newman.

626   **Jeejeebhoy, K. N.** (1988). *Current therapy in nutrition*. Toronto: B. C. Decker. 497 pp.
Discusses and informs the reader about the role of nutrition in the treatment of various disorders; emphasizes brevity and practicality rather than theoretical detail.

*627   **McLaren, D. S.** (1981). *Nutrition and its disorders*. 3rd ed. Edinburgh: Churchill Livingstone. 288 pp.
A textbook primarily for dietetic students, giving a co-ordinated outline of theory and practice of all aspects of nutrition and dietetics.

*628   **Buss, D.** and **Robertson, J.** (1985). *Manual of nutrition*. 9th ed. London: HMSO for the Ministry of Agriculture Fisheries and Food. 144 pp.
Describes all the important nutrients, their functions in the body, digestion and assimilation, effects of cooking on food, special nutritional requirements, and nutrient values; includes relevant UK legislation.

*629   **Nilson, B.** (1981). *Cooking for special diets*. 3rd ed. Harmondsworth, Middx: Penguin. 459 pp.
Of direct interest to dietetic students and the carers of patients discharged from hospital, when a prescribed diet is translated into palatable meals; all the recipes given have been tested.

*630   Pike, R. L. and **Brown, X.** (1984). *Nutrition: an integrated approach.* 3rd ed. New York, NY: John Wiley. 1068 pp.

*631   Shils, M. E. and **Young, V. R.** (1988). *Modern nutrition in health and disease.* 7th ed. Philadelphia, PA: Lea & Febiger. 1694 pp.

*632   Thomas, B. (1988). *Manual of dietetic practice.* Oxford: Blackwell Scientific. 638 pp.
A unique text, designed primarily for qualified and student dietitians but of interest to doctors, medical students and nurses; it is specifically concerned with practical aspects of dietetic care, supplying essential practical details needed to deal with nutrition problems.

*633   Trowell, H., Burkitt, D. and **Heaton, K.**, eds (1985). *Dietary fibre, fibre-depleted food and disease.* London: Academic Press. 433 pp.

Healthy Eating

634   Health Education Authority (1987). *Nutrition education: resource list.* London: HEA. 46 pp.

635   Henley, A. (1982). *Asian patients in hospital and at home.* 2nd ed. London: King Edwards Hospital Fund. 198 pp.
Aims to familiarize readers with the general details of the diets of the main Asian groups in Britain; it comprises a trainer's manual, slides, OHPs and information booklets.

*636   Leverkus, C. *et al.* (1985). *The Great British diet.* London: Century Publishing. 192 pp.
A fascinating insight into the problems of eating for health, and a practical guide for action.

637   Maryon-Davis, A. and **Thomas, J.** (1984). *Diet 2000.* London: Pan. 154 pp.
Healthy eating for individuals and the family; the dietary principles are based on the NACNE recommendations.

Pregnancy and Lactation

*638   Campbell, D. M. and **Gillmer, M. D. G.** (1983). *Nutrition in pregnancy.* London: Royal College of Obstetricians and Gynaecologists.

639   Eiger, M. S. and **Olds, S. W.** (1972). *The complete book of breastfeeding.* New York, NY: Workman Publishing Co. 209 pp.

Readable, helpful coverage of all aspects of breastfeeding from the 'practical mechanics' to the psychological manifestations.

*640   Pickard, B. (1984). *Eating well for a healthy pregnancy.* London: Sheldon Press. 154 pp.
An easy-to-read, practical guide to healthy eating before, during and after pregnancy, giving advice on food choice and guidance about other potential hazards in pregnancy, including alcohol and smoking; covers every aspect of nutrition required by parents-to-be and carers.

*641   Stanway, A. and **Stanway, P.** (1983). *Breast is best.* 2nd ed. London: Pan. 288 pp.
A comprehensive guide explaining how breast feeding works, how to prepare for it and look after the mother's diet and health.

Paediatrics

642   Bampfylde, H. and **Dickerson, J.** (1985). *Healthy eating for your child.* London: Collins. 144 pp.
Combines scientific research and nutritional information with practical advice and easy-to-follow economical recipes, to produce a comprehensive guide on how to feed a child the healthy way.

*643   Bentley, D. and **Lawson, M.** (1988). *Clinical nutrition in paediatric disorders.* London: Baillière Tindall.
Aimed at paediatricians and paediatric nutritionists, this book is in three parts: normal dietary requirements; gastroenterology and hepatic disorders; cardiac and renal disease, diabetes and obesity; useful appendices and references. A very useful reference book for a general hospital dietetic department.

*644   Francis, D. E. M. and **Dixon, D. J. W.** (1986). *Diets for sick children.* 4th ed. Oxford: Blackwell. 422 pp.
Excellent up-to-date text giving practical assistance to medical, nursing and dietetic staff on specialised therapeutic diets for children.

645   Francis, D. E. M. (1986). *Nutrition for children.* Oxford: Blackwell. 176 pp.
Details the nutritional needs of infants and children with tables and guides; a practical guide for feeding children in the 1980s.

646   McLaren, D. and **Burman, D.** (1982). *Textbook of paediatric nutrition.* 2nd ed. Edinburgh: Churchill Livingstone. 464 pp.

647   Walker-Smith, J. A. (1979). *Diseases of the small intestine in childhood.* 2nd ed. London: Pitman. 412 pp.

A nice blend of basic physiology, pathology and practical aspects of diagnosis and treatment.

648   Wharton, B. A. (1980). *Nutrition and feeding of pre-term infants*. Oxford: Blackwell. 250 pp.

649   Wood, C. B. S. and **Walker-Smith, J. A.** (1981). *MacKeith's Infant feeding and feeding difficulties*. 6th ed. Edinburgh: Churchill Livingstone. 334 pp.
A well-known textbook giving practical and topical information on all aspects of infant feeding.

Elderly

*650   Davies, L. (1981). *Three score years . . . and then?* London: Heinemann. 256 pp.

Diabetes

*651   Bloom, A. (1982). *Diabetes explained*. 4th ed. Lancaster: MTP. 168 pp.
Valuable information and practical advice for the diabetic and carer.

652   British Diabetic Association (1988). *Countdown, carbohydrate, calories*. London: British Diabetic Association. 223 pp.
The only book of its kind in the UK, listing over 1000 foods in categories according to nutrient content, sugar, fat, fibre and carbohydrate values 'per serving'; makes countdown a valuable method for diabetics who wish to make an informed choice about everyday foods.

653   Craig, O. (1981). *Childhood diabetes and its management*. 2nd ed. Sevenoaks, Kent: Butterworths. 336 pp.
The author shares his experience and includes useful case histories.

*654   Day, J. L. (1986). *The diabetes handbook: insulin dependent diabetes*. Wellingborough, Northants.: Thorsons. 248 pp.
A clear and simple guide for people with insulin dependent diabetes and their carers, to help them control their blood sugar levels and live their lives to the full. Covers symptoms, control, treatment, keeping the balance, marriage and pregnancy, and diabetes in children.

*655   Day, J. L. (1986). *The diabetes handbook: non-insulin dependent diabetes*. Wellingborough, Northants.: Thorsons. 129 pp.
A similar guide to [654].

*656   Oakley, W., Pyke, D. and **Taylor, K.** (1978). *Diabetes and its management*. 3rd ed. Oxford: Blackwell. 225 pp.

A practical guide to the management of diabetes, including useful basic biochemistry; helpful to those taking higher examinations, answering a lot of questions.

*657   **Sonksen, P., Fox, C.** and **Judd, S.** (1985). *Diabetes reference book*. London: Harper & Row. 295 pp.
A question-and-answer guide, including sections on hypodermics and insulin.

658   **Tattersall, R.** (1986). *Diabetes: a practical guide for patients on insulin*. 2nd ed. Edinburgh: Churchill Livingstone. 196 pp.

*659   **Thomas, B.** (1984). *Diet and diabetes*. Edinburgh: Churchill Livingstone. 97 pp.
A brief but clear description of the dietary factors to be considered in the treatment of diabetes. It also includes recipes and useful tips for recipe adaptation.

*660   **Turner, M.** and **Thomas, B.** (1981). *Nutrition and diabetes*. London: John Libbey. 112 pp.

Renal

*661   **Berlyne, G. M.** (1986). *Nutrition in renal disease*. Edinburgh: Churchill Livingstone. 251 pp.
These proceedings give a valuable exchange of information between professional nutritionists and food manufacturers on the role of nutrition in renal disease.

662   **Cameron, S., Russell, A.** and **Sale, D.** (1976). *Nephrology for nurses*. 2nd ed. London: Heinemann. 330 pp.
All aspects of nephrology are covered concisely.

Gastroenterology

*663   Nutritional support (1988). *Baillière's Clinical Gastroenterology*, **2** (4).
A very important reference on nutritional support in gastrointestinal disorders.

Enteral and Parenteral Nutrition

*664   **Grant, A.** and **Todd, E.** (1987). *Enteral and parenteral nutrition*. 2nd ed. Oxford: Blackwell. 288 pp.
A clinical handbook for all staff involved in nutritional support, providing important data on the optimum regimen for any patient.

*665   **Silk, D. B. A.** (1983). *Nutritional support in hospital practice*. Oxford: Blackwell. 192 pp.

*666   **Wright, R. A.** and **Heymsfield, S.**, eds (1984). *Nutritional assessment.* Oxford: Blackwell. 312 pp.

Mental Health

*667   **Abraham, S.** and **Llewellyn-Jones, D.** (1984). *Eating disorders: the facts.* Oxford: Oxford University Press. 170 pp.

*668   **Bruch, H.** (1974). *Eating disorders: obesity, anorexia and the person within.* London: Routledge & Kegan Paul. 408 pp.

*669   **Melville, J.** (1983). *The ABC of eating: coping with anorexia, bulimia and compulsive eating.* London: Sheldon Press. 112 pp.
Describes the complex reasons for the onset of anorexia, bulimia and compulsive eating and the various types of prescribed treatments.

Obesity

670   **Health Education Authority** (1987). *Obesity: resource list prepared by the Health Education Authority.* London: HEA.

*671   **Garrow, J. S.** (1981). *Treat obesity seriously.* Edinburgh: Churchill Livingstone. 246 pp.
The entire range of obesity problems is presented, the use of diet is reviewed and management options are outlined.

Community

672   **Lennon, D.** and **Fieldhouse, P.** (1979). *Community dietetics.* London: Forbes Publications. 127 pp.

Allergies and Intolerance

*673   **Gray, J.** (1986). *Food intolerance: fact and fiction.* London: Grafton Books. 152 pp.
Designed to explode some myths surrounding food allergies and intolerances.

674   **Hanssen, M.** (1986). *E for additives.* Wellingborough, Northants.: Thorsons. 224 pp.
A comprehensive list of food additives.

Biochemistry and Physiology

675   **Barker, B. M.** and **Bender, D. A.** (1980). *Vitamins in medicine.* London: Heinemann. 2 volumes.

676   James, D. E. (1980). *Introduction to psychology*. London: Granada. 400 pp.
A valuable introduction to the field of psychology which gives the (non-psychologist) professional a working knowledge of the subject.

677   Newsholme, E. A. and **Leach, A. R.** (1983). *Biochemistry for the medical sciences*. Chichester: John Wiley.

Metabolism and Research

*678   Prasad, A. S., ed. (1982). *Clinical, biochemical and nutritional aspects of trace elements*. New York, NY: Alan R. Liss. 598 pp.

*679   Silverstone, T. (1982). *Drugs and appetite*. London: Academic Press. 187 pp.

*680   Underwood, E. J. (1986). *Trace elements in human nutrition*. 5th ed. London: Academic Press. 499 pp.

Food Production

681   Green, S. (1985). *Keyguide to information sources in food science and technology*. London: Mansell. 231 pp.
A useful reference work, listing 766 items.

681a   Health Education Authority (1987). *Food hygiene: resource list*. London: HEA. 21 pp.

682   Pacey, A. and **Payne, P.**, eds (1985). *Agricultural development and nutrition*. London: Hutchinson.

NUTRITION TABLES

A knowledge of the composition of foods is essential in the dietary management and treatment of disease and in most quantitative studies of human nutrition.

*683   Paul, A. A. and **Southgate, D. A. T.** (1978). *McCance and Widdowson's Composition of foods*. 4th ed. London: HMSO. 418 pp.

*683a   Paul, A. A., Southgate, D. A. T. and **Russell, J.** (1980). *Amino acid and fatty acid composition: first supplement to McCance and Widdowson's Composition of foods*. London: HMSO. 113 pp.

*683b   Tan, S. P., Wenlock, R. W. and Buss, D. H. (1985). *Foods used by immigrants in the United Kingdom: second supplement to McCance and Widdowson's Composition of foods*. London: HMSO. 74 pp.

*683c   Holland, B., Unwin, I. and Buss, D. H. (1988). *Cereals and cereal products: third supplement to McCance and Widdowson's Composition of foods*. London: Royal Society of Chemistry and Ministry of Agriculture, Fisheries and Food. 147 pp.

*683d   Holland, B., Unwin, I. and Buss, D. H. (1989). *Milk products and eggs: fourth supplement to McCance and Widdowson's Composition of foods*. London: Royal Society of Chemistry and Ministry of Agriculture, Fisheries and Food. 146 pp.

AUDIO-VISUAL MATERIALS

684   Breast feeding: if you want to, you can. (1980). London: Brilliant Ideas Productions. Video, 60 minutes.
For domestic and trained staff use, prepared with the advice of the Royal College of Midwives and the Health Visitors' Association. An A-to-Z guide to breast feeding from birth to post-natal ward to home; getting out; returning to work; weaning.

685   *Oh what a lovely mess*. (1987). London: Royal Society of Medicine. Video, 17 minutes.
Shows how various mothers successfully coped with weaning and gives their practical suggestions and ideas.

686   *The essential ingredient*. (1988). London: Royal Society of Medicine. Video, 25 minutes.
The role of dietitians today, with people, their diet and health.

687   *Nutrition and modified diet*. (1983). London: DHSS. Mixed media training pack.
A tutor's pack with seven kits to allow flexibility in programming sessions; includes slides and OHPs. An excellent teaching aid.

BRITISH DIETETIC ASSOCIATION PUBLICATIONS

The British Dietetic Association publishes a wide range of books, reports and educational materials, some of which are listed here. A full catalogue can be obtained from the Association's Publications Manager at 7th Floor, Elizabeth House, Suffolk Street, Birmingham B1 1LS, England.

688   Austin, E. (1984). *Handbook of metabolic dietetics*. Birmingham: British Dietetic Association.

689   Bateman, C. (1986). *The history of the British Dietetic Association*. Birmingham: British Dietetic Association.

690   Bond, S. (1983). *The professional approach*. Birmingham: British Dietetic Association. 40 pp.
On freelance work and private practice.

691   British Dietetic Association, Child Health and Nutrition Working Party (1987). *Children's diets and change*. Birmingham: British Dietetic Association.

692   British Dietetic Association, Research Committee (1986). *Getting started on research*. Birmingham: British Dietetic Association.

693   Hanes, F. A. and **De Looy, A. E.** (1987) *Can I afford the diet? A discussion paper*. Birmingham: British Dietetic Association.

REPORTS

694   British Medical Association, Board of Science and Education (1986). *Diet, nutrition and health: a report of the Board. . . .* London: BMA. 69 pp.

695   Cole-Hamilton, I. and **Lang, T.** (1986). *Tightening belts: a report on the impact of poverty on food*. London: London Food Commission. LFC Report no. 13.

696   Commission for Racial Equality (1976). *A guide to Asian diets*. 2nd ed. London: Commission for Racial Equality. 20 pp.

697   Health Education Authority (May 1988). *Look after your heart. Strategy document, phase two*. London: Health Education Authority.

698   Lobstein, T. (1988). *Children's food: the good, the bad and the useless*. London: London Food Commission.

699   Lobstein, T. (1988). *Fast food facts: a survival guide to the good, the bad and the really ugly of fast foods*. London: London Food Commission.

700   London Food Commission (1986). A report of the Food and Black Ethnic Minorities Conference, 6 November 1986. London: London Food Commission. LFC Report no. 16.

701   Miller, M. (1985). *Danger, additives at work: a report on food additives, their use and control*. 2nd ed. London: London Food Commission. 172 pp.

702   National Advisory Committee on Nutrition Education (1983). *A discussion paper on proposals for nutritional guidelines for health education in Britain: the NACNE report*. London: Health Education Council. 40 pp.

703   National Research Council (1985). *Recommended dietary allowances*. 10th revision. Washington, DC: National Academy of Sciences Press.

704   Royal College of Physicians (1983). *Obesity*; report of a Working Party, chairman, Sir Douglas Black. London: Royal College of Physicians. 58 pp.

705   Royal College of Physicians and British Nutrition Foundation (1984). *Food intolerance and food aversion: a joint report*. London: Royal College of Physicians.

706   Sheppard, J. (1987). *The big chill: a report on the implications of cook-chill catering for the public service*. London: London Food Commission. 124 pp.

707   University of Bradford, Food Policy Research Unit. *Food Policy Research Briefing Papers*.

707a   Freckleton, A. (1986). *The impact of a supermarket nutrition information programme*. 39 pp.

707b   Montague, S. (1985). *Healthy eating and the NHS*. 45 pp.

707c   Slattery, J. (1986). *Diet/health: food industry initiatives*. A review of initiatives following the NACNE and COMA reports. 132 pp.

707d   Wheelock, V. (1984). *COMA report: Diet and cardiovascular disease*. 15 pp. See also [718].

707e   Wheelock, V. (1984). *Food additives in perspective*. 124 pp.

708   University of Manchester, Department of Community Medicine, Unit of Continuing Education (1983). *District food policies: issues, problems and opportunities*. Manchester: University of Manchester. 105 pp.

709   Wenlock, R. W. *et al.* (1986). *The diets of British school children*. Preliminary report of a nutritional analysis of a nationwide survey of British school children. London: DHSS Leaflets Unit. 68 pp.

709a   Wenlock, R. W. *et al.* (1989). *The diets of British school children.* Final report. London: HMSO. 293 pp.

710   Food and Agriculture Organization (1985). *Energy and protein requirements.* Geneva: World Health Organization. WHO Technical Report series no. 724.

Education

711   British Nutrition Foundation (1977). *Nutrition education.* Report of a working party of the BNF, DHSS and HEC. London: DHSS. 30 pp.

712   Council for Professions Supplementary to Medicine (1979). *PSM education: the next decade. Higher and further education working report.* London: CPSM.

713   Council for Professions Supplementary to Medicine (1970). *PSM registration and self-regulation: future requirements and opportunities. Report of the working party on the future.* London: CPSM.

714   Macdonald, I. (1975). *Dietitians of the future.* A report by a Working Party of the Dietitians Board. London: CPSM.

Government Publications

715   Artificial feeds for the young infant. Report of the Working Party on the Composition of Foods . . ., chairman J. E. Oppe. (1980). London: HMSO. 104 pp. DHSS Reports on Health and Social Subjects no. 18.

716   Crawley, H. (1988). *Food portion sizes.* A report to the Food Standards Committee of the Ministry of Agriculture Fisheries and Food. London: HMSO. 81 pp.

717   Department of Health and Social Security (1981). *Avoiding heart attacks.* London: HMSO. 72 pp.

718   Department of Health and Social Security, Committee on Medical Aspects of Food Policy (1984). *Diet and cardiovascular disease.* Report of the Panel on Diet in Relation to Cardiovascular Disease, chairman P. J. Randle; 'the COMA Report'. London: HMSO. DHSS Reports on Health and Social Subjects no. 28. 32 pp. See also [707d].

719   Department of Health and Social Security (1988). *Present day practices in infant feeding.* 3rd ed. London: HMSO. 66 pp. DHSS Reports on Health and Social Subjects no. 32.

720   Department of Health and Social Security (1985). *Recommended daily amounts of food energy and nutrients for groups of people in the United Kingdom*. London: HMSO. DHSS Reports on Health and Social Subjects no. 15.

721   Department of Health and Social Security, Committee on Medical Aspects of Food Policy (1988). *Third Report of the Sub-Committee on Nutritional Surveillance, executive summary*, chairman J. S. Garrow. London: HMSO. DHSS Reports on Health and Social Subjects no. 33.

722   Department of Health and Social Security, Committee on Medical Aspects of Food Policy (1987). *The use of very low calorie diets in obesity*. London: HMSO. 52 pp. DHSS Reports on Health and Social Subjects no. 31.

723   Knight, I. and **Eldridge, J.** (1984). *The heights and weights of adults in Great Britain*. London: HMSO. 92 pp. OPCS Report no. 1138.

724   Ministry of Agriculture, Fisheries and Food (1987). *The use of the word 'natural' and its derivatives in the labelling, advertising and presentation of food*. Report of a survey by the Local Authorities Co-ordinating Body on Trading Standards. London: HMSO.

725   Ministry of Agriculture, Fisheries and Food (1987). *Household food consumption and expenditure*. Report of the National Food Survey Committee. London: HMSO. 215 pp.

726   Ministry of Agriculture, Fisheries and Food, Food Sciences Division (1987). *Survey of consumer attitudes to food additives: a report prepared for MAFF*. . . . London: HMSO. Vol. 1, *Reports*, 158 pp. Vol. 2, Computer tabulations, 224 pp.

727   Ministry of Agriculture, Fisheries and Food, Steering Group on Food Surveillance (1988). *The British diet – finding the facts*. Report of the Working Party on Nutrients, chairman W. H. B. Denner. London: HMSO. 36 pp. Food Surveillance Paper no. 23.

728   *Rickets and osteomalacia*. Report of the Working Party on the Fortification of Foods with Vitamin D, chairman E. M. Widdowson. (1980). London: HMSO. DHSS Reports on Health and Social Subjects no. 19.

729   Statutes (1960). Professions Supplementary to Medicine Act 1960. London: HMSO.

6 Speech Therapy

Pat Munro

PERIODICALS

Major periodicals are marked*. All periodicals listed have annual indexes, except *Bulletin of the College of Speech Therapists*.

Speech

*730 *Aphasiology*. London: Taylor & Francis. 6 pa. 1987–. International; academic and clinical studies; book reviews.

731 *ASHA*. Rockville, MD: American Speech–Language–Hearing Association. 12 pa. 1959–.
Articles; reviews of books and materials; news and committee reports; classified advertisements. Cumulated indexes with *Journal of Speech and Hearing Disorders*, *Journal of Speech and Hearing Research*, and *Language, Speech and Hearing Services in Schools*: 1936–1961; 1962–1971; 1972–1981.

732 *Australian Journal of Human Communication Disorders*. East Melbourne, Victoria: Australian Association of Speech and Hearing. 2 pa. 1973–.
Research and clinical articles; reviews of books and materials. Cumulated index 1951–1975 in 1977, **5** (2), 156–69.

*733 *British Journal of Disorders of Communication*. London: Cole & Whurr. 3 pa. 1966–.

Academic journal of the College of Speech Therapists; main British journal for speech therapists; book reviews. Cumulated index 1–5, 1966–1970.

734 *Bulletin, College of Speech Therapists*. London: College of Speech Therapists. 12 pa.

Some articles, but mainly news and announcements; supplement with job advertisements.

*735 *Child Language Teaching and Therapy*. London: Arnold. 3 pa. 1985–.
Articles, including teaching articles relevant to therapists; book reviews.

*736 *Clinical Linguistics and Phonetics*. London: Taylor & Francis. 4 pa. 1987–.
International, academic and clinical; letters; reviews.

*737 *Folia Phoniatrica*. Basel: S. Karger for the International Association of Logopedics and Phoniatrics. 6 pa. 1948–.
International, some articles in French, German, etc. with English abstracts; some news of IALP including abstracts of conference papers; reviews.

738 *Human Communication Canada*. Toronto: Canadian Association of Speech–Language Pathologists and Audiologists. 5 pa. 1973–.
Clinical and research articles; reviews.

739 *Journal of Childhood Communication Disorders*. Arlington, VA: Council for Exceptional Children. 2 pa. 1978–.
Frequently publishes issues on one topic; reviews.

740 *Journal of Communication Disorders*. Amsterdam: Elsevier. 6 pa. 1967–.
Original articles, research and advances in knowledge; occasional reviews; American.

741 *Journal of Fluency Disorders*. Amsterdam: Elsevier. 6 pa. 1976–.
The only journal devoted to stammering; mostly original research articles; occasional reviews.

*742 *Journal of Speech and Hearing Disorders*. Rockville, MD: American Speech–Language–Hearing Association. 4 pa. 1936–.
Nature and treatment of disorders, mainly with clinical applications. Cumulated indexes with *ASHA* [731].

*743 *Journal of Speech and Hearing Research*. Rockville, MD: American Speech–Language–Hearing Association. 4 pa. 1958–.
Studies of processes, experimental reports, review papers. Cumulated indexes with *ASHA* [731].

744 *Journal of Voice.* New York, NY: Raven Press. 4 pa. 1987–.
The official journal of the Voice Foundation (USA) and the only periodical devoted to voice; clinical and research articles on all aspects.

745 *Language and Speech.* Teddington, Middx: Kingston Press Services. 4 pa. 1958–.
Tends to carry rather esoteric material, not always relevant for speech therapists; reviews; mostly American.

746 *Language Speech and Hearing Services in Schools.* Rockville, MD: American Speech–Language–Hearing Association. 4 pa. 1970–.
Although specific, this has many articles useful for speech therapists; good descriptions of tests. Cumulated indexes with *ASHA* [731].

747 *New Zealand Speech–Language Therapists' Journal.* Christchurch: New Zealand Speech–Language Therapists' Association. 2 pa. 1946–.
Articles from many sources, not only NZ; also news.

*748 *Seminars in Speech and Language.* Stuttgart: Thieme. 4 pa. 1980–.
Issues on individual topics with a guest editor, all with clinical relevance.

749 *South African Journal of Communication Disorders.* Braamfontein: South African Speech and Hearing Association. Annual. 1977–.
Theoretical, therapeutic and research articles; some in Afrikaans with English abstracts.

Speech and Language: Advances in Basic Research and Practice [823].

750 *Speech Therapy in Practice.* London: Good Impressions Publishing Co. 12 pa (4 pa until 1989). 1985–.
Up-to-date articles; abstracts; reviews; announcements, letters, job advertisements.

*751 *Topics in Language Disorders.* Rockville, MD: Aspen Press. 4 pa. 1980–.
Issues on separate topics, linking theory with practical applications.

Language and Linguistics

752 *Applied Psycholinguistics: Psychological Studies of Language Processes.* Cambridge: Cambridge University Press. 4 pa. 1980–.
International; includes book reviews.

*753 *Brain and Language.* New York, NY: Academic Press. 6 pa. 1974–.
Concerned with language and communication related to brain function. Research articles, case histories; reviews.

754   *First Language.* Chalfont St Giles, Bucks: Alpha Academic. 3 pa. 1980–.
Articles on child language acquisition and development. Includes reviews.

*755   *Journal of Child Language.* Cambridge: Cambridge University Press. 3
  pa. 1974–.
Articles on scientific study of child language and behaviour; not restricted to
English; includes reviews. Cumulated index 1–10, 1974–1983.

756   *Journal of Linguistics.* Cambridge: Cambridge University Press. 2 pa. 1965–.
Theoretical articles on all aspects of linguistics; reviews.

757   *Journal of Memory and Language.* New York, NY: Academic Press. 6 pa.
  1985–.
Original scientific articles on memory and language processing

758   *Journal of Psycholinguistic Research.* New York, NY: Plenum Press. 6 pa.
  1971–.
Theoretical and experimental papers, surveys and reviews from all relevant
disciplines.

759   *Language and Cognitive Processes.* Hove, W. Sussex: Erlbaum Associates. 4 pa.
  1985–.
International; theoretical and experimental papers, surveys and reviews on the
psychological study of language.

760   *Linguistic Inquiry.* Cambridge, MA: MIT Press. 4 pa. 1970–.
International; research on current topics in linguistic theory.

Audiology

761   *British Association of Teachers of the Deaf Journal.* Luton: BATD. 6 pa.
  1902–.
Members' journal; articles, book reviews; notices of courses, job advertisements.

*762   *British Journal of Audiology.* New York, NY: Academic Press. 4 pa. 1967–.
Official journal of the British Society of Audiology; includes international articles
primarily for specialists and technologists in the field; reports of meetings with
abstracts; book reviews, job advertisements. Cumulated index 7–21, 1973–1987
in 1988, **22** (1), 63–80.

763   *Ear and Hearing.* Baltimore, MD: Williams & Wilkins for the American
  Auditory Society. 6 pa. 1975–.
Current research and new clinical applications in audiology and related fields;
book reviews; calendar of events.

Psychology

764 *British Journal of Clinical Psychology*. Leicester: British Psychological Society. 4 pa. 1981–.

765 *British Journal of Developmental Psychology*. Leicester: British Psychological Society. 4 pa. 1983–.

766 *British Journal of Psychology*. Leicester: British Psychological Society. 4 pa. 1904–.

767 *Cognitive Neuropsychology*. Hove, W. Sussex: Erlbaum Associates. 4 pa. 1984–.

768 *Journal of Child Psychology and Psychiatry*. Oxford: Pergamon Press. 6 pa. 1960–.

769 *Journal of Experimental Child Psychology*. New York, NY: Academic Press. 6 pa. 1964–.

Mental Handicap

770 *American Journal of Mental Deficiency*. Washington, DC: American Association on Mental Retardation. 6 pa. 1876–.

771 *Education and Training in Mental Retardation*. Arlington, VA: Council for Exceptional Children. 4 pa. 1966–.

772 *Journal of Autism and Developmental Disorders*. New York, NY: Plenum Press. 4 pa. 1979–.

773 *Mental Handicap*. Kidderminster, Worcs.: British Institute of Mental Handicap. 4 pa. 1982–.

774 *Mental Retardation*. Washington, DC: American Association on Mental Retardation. 6 pa. 1963–.

Children

775 *Child Care, Health and Development*. Oxford: Blackwell. 6 pa. 1975–.

776 *Child Development*. Chicago, IL: University of Chicago Press for the Society for Research in Child Development. 6 pa. 1930–.

Developmental Medicine and Child Neurology [789].

777   *Early Child Development and Care*. London: Gordon & Breach. 4 issues/volume, 3 or 4 volumes pa. 1971–.

778   *Journal of Developmental and Behavioral Pediatrics*. Baltimore, MD: Williams & Wilkins. 6 pa. 1980–.

Special Education

779   *British Journal of Special Education*, continuation of *Special Education, Forward Trends*. Stratford-upon-Avon: National Council for Special Education. 4 pa. 1985–.
Cumulated index to *Special Education, Forward Trends*, 1974–1983.

780   *Exceptional Children*. Arlington, VA: Council for Exceptional Children. 6 pa. 1934–.

781   *Special Children*. Birmingham: Special Children. 10 pa. 1986–.

Non-vocal Communication

782   *Augmentative and Alternative Communication*. Baltimore, MD: Williams & Wilkins for the International Society for Augmentative and Alternative Communication. 4 pa. 1985–.

783   *Communication Outlook*. Toronto: International Society for Augmentative and Alternative Communication. 4 pa. 1978–.

Medical

784   *Cleft Palate Journal*. Philadelphia, PA: B. C. Decker for the American Cleft Palate Association. 4 pa. 1964–.
Includes *International Craniofacial–Cleft Palate Bibliography* [791], 1985–.

Neurology

785   *Brain*. Oxford: Oxford University Press. 4 pa. 1878–.

786   *Cortex*. Paris: Masson. 4 pa. 1964–.

Gerontology

787   *Age and Ageing*. London: Baillière Tindall for the British Geriatrics Society. 4 pa. 1972–.

CURRENT AWARENESS, ABSTRACTS AND INDEXES

British Institute of Mental Handicap Current Awareness Service [324].

788 *Child Development Abstracts and Bibliography.* Chicago, IL: University of Chicago Press for the Society for Research in Child Development. 3 pa. 1927–. Classified with author and subject indexes; includes book reviews.

789 *Developmental Medicine and Child Neurology.* Oxford: Blackwell. 6 pa. 1962–. Each issue contains an index to current articles and abstracts; supplements, published irregularly, include individual bibliographies of publications in each year, and books and articles on many topics of interest, particularly on disorders of communication and hearing.

790 *DSH Abstracts.* Washington, DC: Deafness Speech and Hearing Publications for ASHA and Gallaudet College. 4 pa. 1–25, 1960–1985. Included books and *c.* 500 international periodicals.

Health Service Abstracts [71].

Hearing (CATS) [76].

791 *International Craniofacial–Cleft Palate Bibliography.* Philadelphia, PA: B. C. Decker for the American Cleft Palate Association. 4 pa. 1968–1984 published separately; published in *Cleft Palate Journal* [784], 1985–. References are gathered by the National Library of Medicine using the *MEDLARS* database; includes papers from *Index Medicus* [58] arranged by subject and author. A section is published in each issue of the journal.

Language and Speech Disorders (CATS) [77].

792 *Linguistics Abstracts.* Oxford: Blackwell. 4 pa. 1985–. Abstracts over 40 periodicals, with author and subject indexes.

793 *Linguistics and Language Behavior Abstracts,* continuation of *Language and Language Behavior Abstracts.* San Diego, CA: Sociological Abstracts Inc. 4 pa. 1967–.

794 *Psycscan.* Washington, DC: American Psychological Association. 4 pa. An abstracted bibliography on Developmental Psychology, Learning and Communication Disorders, Mental Retardation; also cumulated volumes on, for example, Learning and communication disorders 1971–1980.

Rehabilitation Index [80].

Rehabilitation Literature [93].

795 *Royal National Institute for the Deaf, Current Awareness Service.* London: RNID. 12 pa.

In six sections: *Language and speech, Hearing, Education, Medicine, Psychology, Social sciences*; each section contains information on recent books and periodical articles, forthcoming meetings, questions in Parliament etc.

BIBLIOGRAPHIES

International Craniofacial–Cleft Palate Bibliography [791].

796   Shulman, B. B. *et al.* (1986). Child language disorders: an annotated bibliography. *ASHA* (American Speech–Language–Hearing Association), **28** (1), 33–41.

797   Silverman, F. H. (1978). Bibliography of literature pertaining to stuttering in elementary-school children. *Journal of Fluency Disorders*, **3**, 87–101. References on stuttering problems of children between the ages of 5 and 12; literature searched included *Dissertation Abstracts*, *DSH Abstracts*, *Language and Language Behavior Abstracts* and *Psychological Abstracts* and their citations. No date coverage is stated, but examination showed 1910 to be the earliest item.

798   Silverman, F. H. *et al.* (1979). Bibliography of literature pertaining to the onset, development and treatment of stuttering during the preschool years. *Journal of Fluency Disorders*, **4**, 171–203.

Literature searched included that in [797] plus *ERIC* and *MEDLINE*.

BOOKS

Anatomy and Physiology

799   Borden, G. J. and **Harris, K. S.** (1984). *Speech science primer: physiology, acoustics and perception of speech.* 2nd ed. Baltimore, MD: Williams & Wilkins. 320 pp.

800   Pegington, J. (1986). *Clinical anatomy in action.* Vol. 2, *The head and neck.* Edinburgh: Churchill Livingstone. 196 pp.

801   Perkins, W. H. and **Kent, R. D.** (1986). *Textbook of functional anatomy of speech, language and hearing.* London: Taylor & Francis. 420 pp.

Child Development

802   Holt, K. S. (1977). *Developmental paediatrics.* London: Butterworths. 304 pp.

803   Illingworth, R. S. (1987). *The development of the infant and young child*. 9th ed. Edinburgh: Churchill Livingstone. 144 pp.

804   Sheridan, M. D. (1975). *Children's developmental progress from birth to five years; the Stycar sequences*. 3rd ed. Windsor: NFER–Nelson. 111 pp.

Cleft Palate

805   Albery, E. H. *et al.*, eds (1986). *Cleft lip and palate, a team approach*. Bristol: John Wright. 104 pp.

806   Stengelhofen, J., ed. (1989). *Cleft palate: the nature and remediation of communication problems*. Edinburgh: Churchill Livingstone. 208 pp.

Hearing

807   Bamford, J. and **Saunders, E.** (1985). *Hearing impairment, auditory perception and language disability*. London: Arnold. 304 pp.

808   Northern, J. L. and **Downs, M. P.** (1984). *Hearing in children*. 3rd ed. Baltimore, MD: Williams & Wilkins. 382 pp.

809   Katz, J., ed. (1985). *Handbook of clinical audiology*. 3rd ed. Baltimore, MD: Williams & Wilkins. 1144 pp.

Language

810   Abudarham, S., ed. (1987). *Bilingualism and the bilingual; an interdisciplinary approach to pedagogical and remedial issues*. Windsor: NFER–Nelson. 212 pp.

811   Bloom, L. and **Lahey, M.** (1978). *Language development and language disorders*. New York, NY: John Wiley. 685 pp.

812   Lahey, M. (1988). *Language disorders and language development*. rev. ed. London: Macmillan. 500 pp.

813   Fletcher, P. and **Garman, M.**, eds (1986). *Language acquisition*. 2nd ed. Cambridge: Cambridge University Press. 613 pp.

814   Wanner, E. and **Gleitman, L. R.**, eds (1982). *Language acquisition: the state of the art*. Cambridge: Cambridge University Press. 532 pp.

Neurology

815   Espir, M. E. and **Rose, F. C.** (1983). *Basic neurology of speech and language*. 3rd ed. Oxford: Blackwell. 224 pp.

Non-vocal Communication

816   **Enderby, P.**, ed. (1987). *Assistive communication aids for the speech impaired.* Edinburgh: Churchill Livingstone. 160 pp.

817   **Kiernan, C.** *et al.* (1982). *Signs and symbols; a review of literature and survey of the use of non-vocal communication systems.* London: Heinemann. Studies in Education no. 11. 290 pp.

Phonology

818   **Grunwell, P.** (1987). *Clinical phonology.* 2nd ed. London: Croom Helm.

Psycholinguistics

819   **Aitchison, J.** (1983). *The articulate mammal: an introduction to psycholinguistics.* 2nd ed. London: Hutchinson. 288 pp.

820   **Clark, H. H.** and **Clark, E. V.** (1977). *Psychology of language: an introduction to psycholinguistics.* New York, NY: Harcourt Brace Jovanovich. 608 pp.

Research

821   **Shearer, W. M.** (1982). *Research procedures in speech language and hearing.* Baltimore, MD: Williams & Wilkins. 262 pp.

Speech Pathology

822   **Darley, F. L., Aronson, A. E.** and **Brown, J. R.** (1975). *Motor speech disorders.* Philadelphia, PA: Saunders. 305 pp.

823   **Lass, N. J.**, ed. (1979). *Speech and language: advances in basic research and practice.* New York, NY: Academic Press. The latest volume is 11, 1984.

823a   **Lass, N. J.** *et al.*, eds (1988). *Handbook of speech–language pathology and audiology.* Philadelphia, PA: B. C. Decker. 1399 pp.

824   **Rieber, R. W.** and **Brubaker, R. S.**, eds (1966). *Speech pathology: an international study of the science.* Amsterdam: North-Holland.

825   **Travis, L. E.**, ed. (1971). *Handbook of speech pathology and audiology.* New York, NY: Appleton-Century-Crofts. 1312 pp.

826   **Van Riper, C.** and **Emerick, L.** (1984). *Speech correction: an introduction to speech pathology and audiology.* 7th ed. New York, NY: Prentice-Hall. 468 pp.

Speech Therapy

827   Eldridge, M. (1968). *History of the treatment of speech disorders*. Edinburgh: Livingstone.

828   Brown, B. B. (1981). *Speech therapy: principles and practice*. Edinburgh: Churchill Livingstone. 272 pp.

829   Bull, T. R. and **Cook, J. L.** (1976). *Speech therapy and ENT surgery*. Oxford: Blackwell.

830   Emerick, L. L. and **Haynes, W. O.** (1986). *Diagnosis and evaluation in speech pathology*. 3rd ed. New York, NY: Prentice-Hall. 368 pp.

831   Johns, D. F., ed. (1985). *Clinical management of neurogenic communicative disorders*. 2nd ed. Boston, MA: Little, Brown. 342 pp.

832   Warner, J. *et al.* (1984). *Speech therapy: a clinical companion. Notes on clinical practice for students*. Manchester: Manchester University Press. 168 pp.

Winslow Press [1312] publications

833   Cooke, J. and **Williams, D.** (1985). *Working with children's language*. Bicester: Winslow Press. 103 pp.

834   Fawcus, M. *et al.* (1985). *Working with dysphasics*. 2nd ed. Bicester: Winslow Press. 129 pp.

835   Hayhow, R. and **Levy, C.** (1989). *Working with stuttering*. Bicester: Winslow Press.

836   Huskins, S. (1986). *Working with dyspraxics*. Bicester: Winslow Press.

837   Langley, J. (1988). *Working with swallowing disorders*. Bicester: Winslow Press. 116 pp.

838   Martin, S. (1987). *Working with dysphonics*. Bicester: Winslow Press.

839   Robertson, S. and **Thomson, F.** (1986). *Working with dysarthrics*. Bicester: Winslow Press. 98 pp.

Stammering

840   Rustin, L. *et al.*, eds (1987). *Progress in the treatment of fluency disorders*. London: Taylor & Francis. 326 pp.

841   Van Riper, C. (1973). *The treatment of stuttering.* New York, NY: Prentice-Hall. 496 pp.

842   Van Riper, C. (1982). *The nature of stuttering.* 2nd ed. New York, NY: Prentice-Hall. 464 pp.

Statistics

843   Howell, D. C. (1987). *Statistical methods for psychology.* 2nd ed. Boston, MA: Duxbury Press.

Voice

844   Aronson, A. E. (1985). *Clinical voice disorders: an interdisciplinary approach.* 2nd ed. New York, NY: Thieme. 417 pp.

845   Edels, Y., ed. (1983). *Laryngectomy: diagnosis to rehabilitation.* London: Croom Helm. 320 pp.

DICTIONARIES

846   Crystal, D. (1987). *The Cambridge Encyclopedia of language.* Cambridge: Cambridge University Press.

847   Crystal, D. (1985). *A first dictionary of linguistics and phonetics.* 2nd ed. Oxford: Blackwell. 352 pp.

848   Morris, D. W. H. (1988). *A dictionary of speech therapy.* London: Taylor & Francis.
In eight sections with references; many therapists do not approve of this.

849   Nicolosi, L. *et al.* (1988). *Terminology of communication disorders: speech-language–hearing.* 3rd ed. Baltimore, MD: Williams & Wilkins. 350 pp.
Dictionary, with a few helpful explanatory articles including lists of tests.

850   Speech Foundation of America (1961). *Stuttering words: a glossary of the meanings of words and terms used or associated with stuttering and speech pathology.* Memphis, TN: Speech Foundation of America. SFA publication no. 2.

851   Worthington, A. (1985). *Glossary of mental handicap and associated physical disorders.* Privately published.

DIRECTORIES

852   Academy of Aphasia (April 1987). *Membership directory*.
Alphabetical and geographical lists and bye-laws.

853   American Speech–Language–Hearing Association (1987). *Membership directory*. Rockville, MD: ASLHA.
Published every few years.

854   Charities Aid Foundation (1983). *Directory of organisations for the deaf and hard of hearing*. Tonbridge, Kent: Charities Aid Foundation.

855   College of Speech Therapists (1987). *Directory*. London: College of Speech Therapists.
Alphabetical and geographical lists of members; information on CST; lists of useful addresses. Updated every few years.

856   Wiltshire County Council Careers Service (1987). *Compendium of post-16 education and training in residential establishments for handicapped young people*. 2nd ed. Salisbury: WCCCS.
Detailed information on residential establishments offering further education and/or training to young people with handicaps or special needs; indexed.

857   Invalid Children's Aid Nationwide, I Can (1988). *I Can list of educational provision for speech and language disordered children*. 3rd ed. London: I Can.
Annual lists of amendments.

858   Voluntary Organisations Communication and Language, VOCAL (undated). *A problem with speech? Where to get help*. London: VOCAL.
Leaflet listing the organizations that together form VOCAL; revised periodically.

CONFERENCE REPORTS

859   *The American Speech–Language–Hearing Association* holds an annual convention in the USA; abstracts of papers presented appear in the October issue of *ASHA* [731]; complete proceedings are not published.

860   *Child Language Seminars, Proceedings*. An annual meeting of child language researchers, held at a British university each year and proceedings issued from that university; abstracts are published (since 1982) in *First Language* [754].

861   *Clinical Aphasiology, Conference Proceedings*. Annual. 1972-. 1–17, 1972–1987, ed. R. H. Brookshire. Minneapolis, MO: BRK Publishers. 18-, 1988-, ed. T. E. Prescott. London: Cole & Whurr.
Annual conferences held at US locations.

862   *College of Speech Therapists, Conference Reports*. 1945-.
A conference is held every three or four years, and published in various forms; the latest is the ninth, 1987.

863   *International Association of Logopedics and Phoniatrics, Congress Proceedings*. 1926-.
A congress is held every three years; the latest is the twentieth, 1986.

ASSESSMENTS, TESTS AND PROGRAMMES

864   **Buros, O. K.**, ed. (1978). *Mental measurements yearbook*. 8th ed. Lincoln, NE: University of Nebraska Press. 2 volumes.

865   **Rustin, L.** (1987). *Assessment and therapy programme for dysfluent children*. Windsor: NFER–Nelson.
Manual, audio cassette, children's workbooks, parents' workbooks, assessment booklets.

866   **Goodglass, H.** and **Kaplan, E.** (1983). *Assessment of aphasia and related disorders*. 2nd ed. Boston, MA: Lea & Febiger.
Boston diagnostic aphasia examination. The test also comprises stimulus cards and scoring booklets; in the 2nd ed. there is also the Boston Naming Test with its scoring booklet.

867   **Anthony, A.** *et al.* (1971). *Edinburgh articulation test*. Edinburgh: Churchill Livingstone.
Textbook, picture book, qualitative assessment sheet, quantitative assessment sheet.

868   **Crystal, D., Fletcher, P.** and **Garman, M.** (1989). *Grammatical analysis of language disability*. 2nd ed. London: Cole & Whurr. (1st ed. was published by Edward Arnold, 1976).
Language assessment remediation and screening procedure. LARSP. Charts are available separately from P O Box 5, Holyhead, Gwynedd LL65 1RG, Wales.

869   **Reynell, J.** (1985). *Reynell developmental language scales*. 2nd ed. Windsor: NFER–Nelson.
Manual, case of toys and other items, record form.

GOVERNMENT REPORTS

870   **Department of Education and Science** (1972). *Speech therapy services*. Report of the Committee . . . 1969, chairman Prof. R. Quirk. London: HMSO. 90 pp.

871   **Department of Education and Science** (1975). *A language for life*. Report of the Committee of Inquiry . . ., chairman Sir Alan Bullock. London: HMSO. 646 pp.

872   **Department of Education and Science** (1978). *Special educational needs*. Report of the Committee of Enquiry into the Education of Handicapped Children and Young People, chairman H. M. Warnock. Cmnd 7212. London: HMSO. 416 pp.

7 Radiography, Diagnostic and Therapeutic

Linda Castleton and Mary Lovegrove

PERIODICALS

873 *Atom: Journal of the UKAEA*. London: United Kingdom Atomic Energy Authority. 12 pa. 1956–.
Includes items on nuclear physics and associated areas.

874 *British Journal of Radiology*. London: Butterworths for the British Institute of Radiology. 12 pa. 1896–.
Covers the entire range of radiological disciplines, including radiodiagnosis, radiotherapy, nuclear medicine, ultrasound, MRI and radiobiology.

875 *Canadian Association of Radiologists, Journal*. Montreal: Canadian Association of Radiologists. 4 pa. 1973–.

876 *Cancer*. Philadelphia, PA: J. B. Lippincott for the American Cancer Society. 12 pa. 1947–.

877 *Clinical Radiology*. Oxford: Blackwell Scientific for the College of Radiologists. 6 pa. 1950–.

878 *Electromedica*. Erlangen, FR Germany: Siemens Verlag AG. 4 pa. 1932–.
Covers the latest developments in imaging technology; in four language editions, English, French, German and Spanish.

879 *International Journal of Radiation: Oncology, Biology and Physics*. Oxford: Pergamon Press. 12 pa. 1976–.
Excellent on all the subjects in the title.

880 *Journal of Clinical Ultrasound*. New York: John Wiley. 6 pa. 1972–.

881 *Rad Magazine*. Harlow, Essex: Kingsmoor Publications. 12 pa. 1975–.
Distributed free of charge to imaging, radiotherapy and medical physics departments.

882 *Radiography Today*. London: College of Radiographers. 12 pa. 1935–.
Covers all subjects related to the entire range of disciplines in radiography, aimed specifically at radiographers.

883 *Radiologic Technology*. Baltimore: Williams & Wilkins for the American Society of Radiologic Technologists. 6 pa. 1929–.

884 *Seminars in Oncology*. Orlando, FL: Grune & Stratton. 4 pa. 1974–.

885 *Seminars in Roentgenology*. Orlando, FL: Grune & Stratton. 4 pa. 1966–.
An excellent review journal, as are [884]iand [886].

886 *Seminars in Ultrasound, CT and MR*. Orlando, FL: Grune & Stratton. 4 pa. 1980–.

BOOKS

Anatomy, Physiology and Pathology

887 **Amos, W. M. G.** (1981). *Basic immunology*. London: Butterworths. 192 pp.

888 **Bloomfield, J. A.** (1982). *Pathology for radiographers and allied health professionals*. Chicago, IL: Year Book Medical Publishers. 150 pp.

889 **Bo, W. J.** *et al.* (1990). *Basic atlas of cross sectional anatomy with correlated imaging*. 2nd ed. Philadelphia, PA: W. B. Saunders 380. pp.
Excellent reproductions of cadaver sections with corresponding ultrasound, computed tomography and magnetic resonance images.

890 **Brown, M.** (1987). *Anatomy, physiology and pathology*. London: Heinemann Medical. 208 pp.
A multiple-choice tutor, published in conjunction with the College of Radiographers, the examining body.

891   Bryan, G. J. (1982). *Johnson and Kennedy's Radiographic skeletal anatomy*. 2nd ed. Edinburgh: Churchill Livingstone. 316 pp.

892   Unused.

893   Dean, M. R. E. and **West, T. E. T.** (1987) *Basic anatomy and physiology for radiographers*. 3rd ed. Oxford: Blackwell Scientific. 528 pp.
Recommended for basic information and good line diagrams.

894   Gunn, C. (1984). *Bones and joints*. Edinburgh: Churchill Livingstone. 188 pp.
Excellent line diagrams together with some tabulated information.

895   Guyton, A. C. (1987). *Human physiology and mechanisms of disease*. 4th ed. Philadelphia, PA: W. B. Saunders. 720 pp.
Student edition also available; highly recommended for all levels of study.

896   Guyton, A. C. (1984). *Physiology of the human body*. 6th ed. Philadelphia, PA: W. B. Saunders. 704 pp.
Clear explanation of in-depth information.

897   Keogh, B. and **Ebbs, S.** (1986). *Normal surface anatomy*. London: Heinemann Medical. 288 pp.
Student edition: comprehensive and well illustrated.

898   Ledley, R. S., Huang, H. K. and **Massiotta, J. C.** (1977). *Cross-sectional anatomy: an atlas for computerized tomography*. Baltimore, MD: Williams & Wilkins. 330 pp.

899   McKears, D. W. and **Owen, R. H.** (1979). *Surface anatomy for radiographers*. Bristol: John Wright. 124 pp.

900   Prime, N. (1987). *Introduction to pathology for radiographers*. New York: Harper & Row. 256 pp.

901   Thomson, A. D. and **Cotton, R. E.** (1983). *Lecture notes on pathology*. 3rd ed. Oxford: Blackwell Scientific. 763 pp.
Highly recommended.

902   Tortora, G. J. and **Anagnostakos, N. P.** (1986). *Principles of anatomy and physiology*. 5th ed. New York: Harper & Row. 764 pp.
Widely used by radiography training establishments as a course textbook.

903 Weir, J. and **Abrahams, P.** (1978). *An atlas of radiological anatomy.*
Tunbridge Wells, Kent: Pitman Medical.
Large, good quality radiographs with complementary line diagrams; recommended for self-instruction; out of print.

904 Westacott, S. and **Hall, J. R. W.** (1988). *Key anatomy for radiology.* London:
Heinemann. 288 pp.
Emphasizes sectional approach to anatomy.

905 Woolf, N. (1986). *Cell, tissue and disease: the basis of pathology.* 2nd ed.
London: Baillière Tindall. 512 pp.
Recommended.

Physics of Radiation and Radiography

906 Aird, E. G. A. (1988). *Basic physics for medical imaging.* London: Heinemann
Medical. 248 pp.
Useful introduction to scientific aspects of medical imaging.

907 Curry, T. S., Dowdey, J. E. and **Murry, R. C.** (1984). *Christensen's Introduction to the physics of diagnostic radiology.* 3rd ed. Philadelphia, PA: Lea &
Febiger. 503 pp.
An excellent text for the advanced student.

908 Dendy, R. P. and **Heaton, B.** (1987). *Physics for radiologists.* 403 pp.
Recommended text covering radiation physics and related principles.

909 Gifford, D. A. (1984). *Handbook of physics for radiologists and radiographers.*
Chichester: John Wiley. 561 pp.
Particularly useful for training schools.

910 National Radiological Protection Board, Health and Safety Executive
(1988). *Guidance notes for the protection of persons against ionising radiations arising from
medical and dental use.* London: NRPB. 87 pp.
An essential purchase for all involved with radiation.

911 Jaundrell-Thompson, F. and **Ashworth, W. J.** (1970). *X-Ray physics and
equipment.* 2nd ed. Oxford: Blackwell Scientific. 786 pp.
Reference book for training schools.

912 Meredith, W. J. and **Massey, J. B.** (1972). *Fundamental physics of radiology.*
2nd ed. Bristol: John Wright. 642 pp.
Useful reference book.

913   Wells, P. N. T. (1982). *Scientific basis of medical imaging.* Edinburgh: Churchill Livingstone. 296 pp.
Useful reference.

914   Wilks, R. J. (1987). *Principles of radiological physics.* 2nd ed. Edinburgh: Churchill Livingstone. 292 pp.
Recommended text for student radiographers at all levels.

Physics of Ultrasound

915   Evans, D. H. *et al.* (1989). *Doppler ultrasound physics, instrumentation and clinical applications.* Chichester, W. Sussex: John Wiley. 281 pp.
Thorough coverage of this topic.

916   Himes, D. L., Hendrick, W. R. and **Starchman, D. E.** (1984). *Ultrasound physics and instrumentation.* Edinburgh: Churchill Livingstone. 212 pp.
Useful text covering basic principles.

917   Hussey, M. (1985). *Basic physics and technology of medical diagnostic ultrasound.* London: Macmillan. 231 pp.
Very superficial coverage.

918   Kremkau, F. W. (1989). *Diagnostic ultrasound: principles, instruments and exercises.* 3rd ed. Philadelphia, PA: W. B. Saunders. 315 pp.
Essential text for all students of medical ultrasound.

919   McDicken, W. N. (1981). *Diagnostic ultrasonics: principles and the use of instruments.* 2nd ed. Chichester, W. Sussex: John Wiley. 359 pp.
Excellent text, but lacking in up-to-date developments.

920   Powis, R. L. and **Powis, W. J.** (1984). *Thinker's guide to ultrasonic imaging.* Baltimore, MD: Urban & Schwarzenberg. 413 pp.
Excellent coverage of scan converter functions.

Patient Care and Hospital Practice

921   Betts-Symonds, G. W. (1984). *Fracture care and management for students.* London: Macmillan. 294 pp.

922   Booth, J. A. (1983). *Handbook of investigations.* New York: Harper & Row. 134 pp. Lippincott Nursing series.
A basic introduction to the subject.

923   Capra, L. G. (1986). *Care of the cancer patient.* 2nd ed. Basingstoke: Macmillan Educational. 476 pp.

Highly recommended for those professionals with little experience in this field.

924   Chandler, M. (1988). *Behind the mask.* Stoke-on-Trent: Change Publications. 76 pp.
A patient's first-hand view of receiving radiotherapy.

925   Chesney, D. N. and **Chesney, M. O.** (1986). *Care of the patient in diagnostic radiography.* 6th ed. Oxford: Blackwell Scientific. 368 pp.
Useful for those involved in therapeutic radiography as well, despite the title.

926   Chesney, D. N. and **Chesney, M. O.** (1986). *A radiographer's handbook of hospital practice.* Oxford: Blackwell Scientific. 142 pp.

927   Ehrlich, R. A. and **McCloskey, E. D.** (1989). *Patient care in radiography.* 3rd ed. St Louis, MO: C. V. Mosby. 298 pp.

928   Gunn, C. and **Tozer, C. S.** (1982). *Guidelines on patient care in radiography.* Edinburgh: Churchill Livingstone. 179 pp.
The tabulated format makes this text easy to use; particularly useful for student radiographers.

929   Hegarty, J. R. and **DeCann, R. W.** (1986). *Psychology in radiography.* Stoke-on-Trent: Change Publications. 150 pp.

930   Hegarty, J. R. and **DeCann, R. W.** (1988). *Psychology in radiography, 2.* Stoke-on-Trent: Change Publications. 150 pp.

931   Neuberger, J. (1987). *Caring for dying people of different faiths.* London: Austen Cornish. 59 pp. Lisa Sainsbury Foundation Series.

932   Saunders, C. M., Summers, D. H. and **Teller, N.** (1981). *Hospice: the living idea.* London: Edward Arnold. 208 pp.
A must for those interested in this field.

933   Open University, U.205 Course Team (1983). *Experiencing and explaining disease.* Milton Keynes: Open University Press. 135 pp.
The recommended text for the second level of the OU's Health and Disease course.

Diagnostic Imaging

934   Bentley, H. B. (1986). *Textbook of radiographic science.* Edinburgh: Churchill Livingstone. 210 pp.
Essential reference for all post-diplomate students.

935   Bryan, G. J. (1987). *Diagnostic radiography: a concise practical manual.* Edinburgh: Churchill Livingstone. 417 pp.
An excellent general text.

936   Chalmers, A. G., McKillop, J. H. and **Robinson, P.J. A.** (1988). *Imaging in clinical practice.* London: Edward Arnold. 330 pp.
Excellent clinical coverage, ideal for reference.

937   Chapman, S. and **Nakielny, R.** (1986). *A guide to radiological procedures.* London: Baillière Tindall. 268 pp.
All copies are well thumbed.

938   Swallow, R. A. *et al.* (1989). *Clark's Positioning in radiography.* Oxford: Heinemann. 418 pp.
Essential textbook.

939   Doyle, T. *et al.* (1989). *Procedures in diagnostic radiology.* Edinburgh: Churchill Livingstone. 228 pp.

940   Evans, K. T. *et al.* (1987). *Clinical radiology for medical students.* London: Butterworths. 136 pp.
Excellent-quality image reproduction.

941   Sider, L. (1986). *Introduction to diagnostic imaging.* Edinburgh: Churchill Livingstone. 290 pp.
Useful detailed reference.

942   Steiner, R. E. and **Sherwood, T.** (1986). *Recent advances in radiology and medical imaging.* Edinburgh: Churchill Livingstone. 208 pp.
Very useful reference.

943   Sutton, D. (1988). *Radiology and imaging for medical students.* Edinburgh: Churchill Livingstone. 244 pp.
Good coverage of the subject.

944   Whitehouse, G. H. and **Worthington, B. S.** (1983). *Techniques in diagnostic radiography.* Oxford: Blackwell Scientific. 351 pp.
Useful reference book.

945   Grech, P. (1981). *Casualty radiology: a practical guide for radiological diagnosis.* London: Chapman & Hall. 238 pp.
Essential reference.

Special and Regional Imaging

946   Bull, S. (1985). *Skeletal radiography*. London: Butterworths. 213 pp.
Good comprehensive text.

947   Griffiths, H. (1981). *Basic bone radiology*. Philadelphia, PA: Appleton-Century-Crofts. 182 pp.
Very useful reference text.

948   Smith, N. J. D. (1980). *Dental radiography*. Oxford: Blackwell Scientific. 126 pp.
Still the best text available.

949   Kimber, P. M. (1983). *Radiography of the head*. Edinburgh: Churchill Livingstone. 197 pp.
The only specialized book of its kind – essential reading.

950   Watkins, P. R. (1984). *A practical guide to chest imaging*. Edinburgh: Churchill Livingstone.
Useful, clearly presented text.

Imaging Techniques

951   Brooker, M. J. (1986). *Computed tomography for radiographers*. Lancaster: MTP Press. 126 pp.
Useful reference for radiographers.

952   Dixon, A. K. (1983). *Body CT: a handbook*. Edinburgh: Churchill Livingstone. 164 pp.
Easy reference.

953   Husband, J. E. and **Fry, I. K.** (1983). *Computed tomography of the body: a radiological and clinical approach*. London: Macmillan. 217 pp.
Useful text from the recognized experts in this field.

954   Kean, D. and **Smith, M.** (1986). *Magnetic resonance imaging*. Over Wallop, Hants.: BAS Printers. 161 pp.
Good coverage of the latest imaging modality.

955   Ell, P. J. and **Williams, E. S.** (1981). *Nuclear medicine: an introductory text*. Oxford: Blackwell Scientific. 200 pp.
Still a useful first text.

956   **Maisey, M. N., Britton, K. E.** and **Gilday, D. L.** (1985). *Clinical nuclear medicine*. Philadelphia, PA: W. B. Saunders. 317 pp.
First class reference.

957   **Chudleigh, P.** and **Pearce, J. M.** (1986). *Obstetric ultrasound: how, why and when*. Edinburgh: Churchill Livingstone. 186 pp.
Essential text for all involved in obstetric scanning.

958   **Cosgrove, D. O.** and **McCready, V. R.** (1983). *Ultrasound imaging: liver, spleen, pancreas*. Chichester, W. Sussex: John Wiley. 363 pp.
Excellent reference.

959   **Grant, E. G.** and **White, E. M.** (1989). *Duplex sonography*. New York: Springer. 259 pp.
Excellent reference for all with an interest in ultrasound.

960   **Saunders, R. C.** (1984). *Clinical sonography: a practical guide*. Boston, MA: Little, Brown & Co. 384 pp.
The standard text.

Oncology and Radiotherapy

961   **Baum, M.** (1988). *Breast cancer: the facts*. Oxford: Oxford University Press. 136 pp.
Useful information for students and the general public.

962   **Cahoon, M. C.**, ed. (1982). *Cancer nursing*. Edinburgh: Churchill Livingstone. 172 pp.

963   **Calnan, J. S.** (1984). *Talking with patients: a guide to good practice*. London: Heinemann Medical. 192 pp.

964   **Carter, S. K., Bakowski, M. T.** and **Hellmann, K.** (1981). *Chemotherapy of cancer*. 2nd ed. Chichester: John Wiley. 379 pp.

965   **Coggle, J. E.** (1983). *Biological effects of radiation*. 2nd ed. London: Taylor & Francis. 247 pp.

966   **Consumers' Association** (1986). *Understanding cancer*. London: Edward Arnold. 160 pp.

967   **Cooper, J. S.** and **Pizzarello, D. J.** (1980). *Concepts in cancer care*. Philadelphia, PA: Lea & Febiger. 273 pp.

968   Deeley, T. J., ed. (1972). *Computers in radiotherapy: clinical aspects*. London: Butterworths. 113 pp.

969   Deeley, T. J., ed. (1982). *Topical reviews in radiotherapy:* volume 2. Bristol: John Wright. 254 pp.

970   DeVita, V. T., Hellman, S. and **Rosenberg, S. A.** (1989). *Principles and practice of oncology*. 3rd ed. Philadelphia, PA: J. B. Lippincott. 2656 pp.
Comprehensive, of value to radiotherapists and teachers.

971   Dobbs, J. and **Barrett, A.** (1985). *Practical radiotherapy planning*. London: Edward Arnold. 248 pp.

972   Doll, R. and **Peto, R.** (1981). *The causes of cancer*. Oxford: Oxford Medical Publishers. 115 pp.
Authoritative text, by internationally recognized epidemiologists.

973   Easson, E. C. and **Pointon, R. C. S.** (1985). *The radiotherapy of malignant disease*. Berlin: Springer-Verlag. 474 pp.

974   Fowler, J. F. (1981). *Nuclear particles in cancer treatment*. Bristol: Adam Hilger. 178 pp. Medical Physics Handbooks series.

975   Greene, D. (1986). *Linear accelerators for radiation therapy*. Bristol: Adam Hilger. 194 pp. Medical Physics Handbooks series.

976   Hancock, B. W. and **Bradshaw, J. D.** (1981). *Lecture notes on clinical oncology*. Oxford: Blackwell Scientific. 215 pp.

977   Unused.

978   Hope-Stone, H. F., ed. (1986). *Radiotherapy in clinical practice*. London: Butterworths. 464 pp.

979   Latham, J. (1987). *Pain control*. London: Austen Cornish. 106 pp. Lisa Sainsbury Foundation series.
Excellent and easy to understand.

980   Levitt, S. H. and **Tapley, N. du V.** (1984). *Technological basis of radiation therapy: practical clinical applications*. Philadelphia, PA: Lea & Febiger. 336 pp.

981   Lochhead, J. N. M. (1983). *Care of the patient in radiotherapy*. Oxford: Blackwell Scientific. 178 pp.

982   Magrath, I., ed. (1989). *New directions in cancer treatment.* Berlin: Springer-Verlag. 629 pp.

983   Moorey, S. and **Greer, S.** (1989). *Psychological therapy for patients with cancer: a new approach.* London: Heinemann Medical. 233 pp.

984   Mould, R. F. (1985). *Brachytherapy 1984: proceedings of the 3rd International Selectron Users Meeting.* Leersum, Netherlands: Nucletron Trading BV. 306 pp.

985   Nias, A. H. W. (1988). *Clinical radiobiology.* 2nd ed. Edinburgh: Churchill Livingstone. 279 pp.

986   Pizzarello, D. J. and **Witkofski, R. L.** (1975). *Basic radiation biology.* 2nd ed. Philadelphia, PA: Lea & Febiger. 143 pp.

987   Pizzarello, D. J. and **Witkofski, R. L.** (1982). *Medical radiation biology.* 2nd ed. Philadelphia, PA: Lea & Febiger. 164 pp.

988   Priestman, T. J. (1977). *Cancer chemotherapy: an introduction.* London: Farmitalia Carlo Erba. 231 pp.

989   Rubin, P. R., ed. (1983). *Clinical oncology.* 6th ed. Rochester, MD: American Cancer Society. 536 pp.

990   Saunders, C. M., ed. (1984). *The management of terminal malignant disease.* London: Edward Arnold. 266 pp.
Management of Malignant Disease series, no. 1.

991   Scott, Sir R. B. (1979). *Cancer: the facts.* Oxford: Oxford Medical Publications. 208 pp.
Useful information for students and the general public.

992   Sikora, K. and **Halnan, K. E.** (1989). *Treatment of cancer.* 2nd ed. London: Chapman & Hall. 912 pp.
Wide-ranging information, of great value to all professionals associated with radiotherapy.

993   Sikora, K. and **Smedley, H.** (1988). *Cancer.* London: Heinemann Medical. 144 pp. Heinemann Student Reviews series.

994   Souhami, R. and **Tobias, J.** (1989). *Cancer and its management.* Oxford: Blackwell Scientific. 526 pp.

995   Steele, G. G., Adams, G. E. and **Peckham, M. J.** (1983). *The biological basis of radiotherapy.* Amsterdam: Elsevier. 336 pp.

996   Stoll, B. A., ed. (1979). *Mind and cancer prognosis*. Chichester, W. Sussex: John Wiley. 203 pp.

997   Taylor, J. (1988). *Imaging in radiotherapy*. London: Croom Helm. 205 pp. Probably the only text dedicated to the application of this subject in this particular field.

998   Tannock, I. F. and **Hill, R. P.** (1987). *The basic science of oncology*. Oxford: Pergamon Press. 398 pp.

999   Tiffany, R. (1978). *Cancer nursing: radiotherapy*. London: Faber. 127 pp.

1000   Tiffany, R. (1978). *Cancer nursing: medical*. London: Faber. 190 pp.

1001   Tiffany, R. (1980). *Cancer nursing: surgical*. London: Faber. 267 pp.

1002   Tiffany, R. (1981). *Cancer nursing update*. London: Baillière Tindall. 200 pp.

1003   Tiffany, R. Oncology for Nurses and Health Care Professionals series. London: Harper & Row. Vol. 1 (1978). *Pathology, diagnosis and treatment*. 332 pp. Vol. 2 (1978). *Care and support*. 255 pp. Vol. 3 (1989). *Cancer nursing*. 256 pp.

1004   Tschudin, V., ed. (1989). *Nursing the patient with cancer*. New York: Prentice-Hall. 512 pp.

1005   Twycross, R. G. and **Lack, S. A.** (1984). *Therapeutics in terminal cancer*. Edinburgh: Churchill Livingstone. 207 pp.

1006   Union Internationale Contre le Cancer (UICC) (1987). *Manual of adult and paediatric medical oncology*. Berlin: Springer-Verlag. 401 pp. Internationally recognized information.

1007   UICC (1982). *TNM atlas: illustrated guide to the classification of malignant tumours*. Berlin: Springer-Verlag. 229 pp. Internationally agreed reference book.

1008   UICC (1987). *TNM classification of malignant tumours*. 4th ed. Berlin: Springer-Verlag. 197 pp. Internationally agreed reference book.

1009   Walter, J., Miller, H. and **Bomford, C. K.** (1979). *A short textbook of radiotherapy*. 4th ed. Edinburgh: Churchill Livingstone. 299 pp. Currently in wide use as a standard student text.

1010   Williams, C. (1984). *Lung cancer: the facts*. Oxford: Oxford University Press. 148 pp.
Suitable for students and the general public.

1011   Williams, C. J. and **Whitehouse, J. M. A.**, eds (1982). *Recent advances in clinical oncology*, no. 1. Edinburgh: Churchill Livingstone. 405 pp.

1012   Williams, C. J. and **Whitehouse, J. M. A.**, eds (1986). *Recent advances in clinical oncology*, no. 2. Edinburgh: Churchill Livingstone. 256 pp.

PART III

List of Selected Organizations

Entries appear at the *first* appropriate point, and are not repeated.

List of Selected Organizations

1   INTERNATIONAL ASSOCIATIONS AND SOCIETIES

Further information on societies is given in Zeitak and Berman's *Directory of . . . medical and related societies* [168].

Chiropody

1013   *Association Européenne des Podologues*, (Madame G. Demoulin, Secretary), Avenue des Cormorans 5, 1150 Bruxelles, Belgium.

1014   *Fédération International de Podologie*, (Secretary, M. Aebi), 13 Rue du Rhône, 1204 Geneva, Switzerland.

Occupational Therapy

1015   *International Society for Prosthetics and Orthotics (UK)*, National Centre for Training and Education in Prosthetics and Orthotics, Curran Building, University of Strathclyde, 131 St James' Road, Glasgow G4 0LS, Scotland.
A multidisciplinary society with national and international meetings. Membership is open to any therapist working in the field, with meetings for presenting research papers and exchange of experience.

1016   *World Federation of Occupational Therapists*, (Hon. Secretary, Mrs B. Posthuma), Department of Occupational Therapy, Health Sciences Center,

University of Western Ontario, London, Ontario, Canada N6A 5C1, *or* contact WFOT delegate at the College of Occupational Therapists [1056].
An international congress is held every four years, and proceedings are published [419].

Physiotherapy

1017   *World Confederation for Physical Therapy*, 16–19 Eastcastle Street, London W1N 7PA, England.

Dietetics

1018   *International Committee for Dietetic Associations*, (Dr J. M. Woodhill), 6/18 St Luke's Road, Randwich, NSW 2031, Australia.

1019   *International Society for Parenteral Nutrition*, (Dr J. M. Long), Department of Surgery, University of Texas Medical School, Houston, TX 77030, USA.

Speech Therapy

1020   *International Association of Logopedics and Phoniatrics*, Avenue de la Gare 6, 1003 Lausanne, Switzerland.

Radiography

1021   *International Society for Radiographers and Radiological Technicians*, 159 Gabalfa Avenue, Cardiff CF4 2PB, Wales.

2   NATIONAL PROFESSIONAL SOCIETIES

Further lists of associations and societies can be found in Zeitak and Berman's *Directory of . . . medical and related societies* [168], Henderson and Henderson's *Directory of British associations* [160], and Darnbrough and Kinrade's *Directory for disabled people* [153].

Allied Health, Paramedical in General

1022   *American Medical Association*, CAHEA, 535 N. Dearborn Avenue, Chicago, IL 60610, USA.

1023   *American Society of Allied Health Professions*, Suite 700, 1101 Connecticut Avenue NW, Washington, DC 20036, USA.

1024   *Association of Professions for the Mentally Handicapped*, Greytree Lodge, Second Avenue, Greytree, Ross-on-Wye, Herefordshire HR9 7EG, England.

1024a *National Association of Health Authorities of England and Wales (NAHA)*, 47 Edgbaston Park Road, Birmingham B15 2RS, England.

Chiropody

1025 *American Podiatric Medical Association*, 9312 Old Georgetown Road, Bethesda, MD 20814–1621, USA.

1026 *Association Belge des Podologues*, (Madame S. Charlier, Secretary), 97 Avenue Crockaert, 1150 Bruxelles, Belgium.

1027 *Association of Chief Chiropody Officers*, 3 New Road, Aston Clinton, Aylesbury, Buckinghamshire HP22 5JD, England.

1028 *Associazone Italiana Podologi*, Via Toscolona 713, 00174 Roma, Italy.

1029 *Associazone Nazionale Italiana Podologi*, Via Ramazzine 3, 20129 Milano, Italy.

1030 *Association of Chiropody Teachers in the UK (ACTUK)*, c/o 2 Vale View Crescent, Llandough, Penarth, South Glamorgan CF6 1NZ, Wales.

1031 *Australian Podiatry Council*, Suite 26, 456 St Kilda Road, Melbourne, Victoria 3004, Australia.

1032 *British Health Professionals in Rheumatology*, c/o Maxton, Higham Road, Tuddenham St Mary, Suffolk IP28 6SG, England.

1033 *British College of Podiatry and Ambulatory Foot Surgeons*, (Mr J. R. Golding), The Surgery, Bay Road, Bracknell, Berkshire RG12 2NR, England.

1034 *British Orthopaedic Foot Society*, (Prof. L. Klenerman), University Dept of Orthopaedic and Accident Surgery, PO Box 147, Royal Liverpool Hospital, Prescot Street, Liverpool L69 3BX, England.

Chiropody Students Association, *Society of Chiropodists* [1043].

District and Area Chiropodists Group, *Society of Chiropodists* [1043].

1035 *Fédération Nationale des Podologues*, 163 Rue Saint-Honoré, 75001 Paris, France.

1036 *Head of Schools of Chiropody Association*, c/o Edinburgh School of Chiropody, Clerwood Terrace, Edinburgh EH12 8TS, Scotland.

Hospital Chiropodists Group, *Society of Chiropodists* [1043].

1037   *Institute of Chiropodists*, 91 Lord Street, Southport, Merseyside PR8 1SA, England.

1038   *Landsforenigen af Stat. Fodterapeuter*, Bjelkees Alle 43, 2200 København, Denmark.

1039   *Nederlande Vereniging van Podotherapeuten*, Postbus 32 58, 5203 DG 's Hertogenbosch, Netherlands.

1040   *New Zealand Society of Podiatrists*, 8 Witham Street, Island Bay, Wellington, New Zealand.

1041   *Podiatry Association*, c/o Secretary, Swaynes Cottage, Fore Street, Weston, near Hitchin, Hertfordshire SG4 7AS, England.

1042   *Schweizerischer Podologen Verband*, Weisse Gasse 15, 4002 Basel, Switzerland.

1043   *Society of Chiropodists*, 53 Welbeck Street, London W1M 7HE, England.

1044   *Society of Chiropodists of Ireland*, 44 Annaville Park, Dundrum Road, Dublin 14, Eire.

1045   *Society of Shoefitters*, Farley Court, Farley Hill, Reading, Berkshire RG7 1TT, England.

1046   *Suomen Jalkojenhoitajain Liito RY*, Ludvigin Katu 7B.7, 00130 Helsinki 13, Finland.

1047   *Sveriges Fotterapeuters Riksforbund*, Regementsgatan 11, 831 41 Östersund, Sweden.

Surgical Interest Group, *Society of Chiropodists* [1043]

1048   *Union des Associations Romandes des Pédicures*, 23 Rue du Grand Pré, 1202 Geneva, Switzerland.

1049   *Verband Österreichischer Fusspfleger*, Kaigasse 32, 5030 Salzburg, Austria.

1050   *Zentralverband der Fusspfleger Deutschlands*, Urgingerstrasse 22, 4130 Moers am Rhein, FRG.

Occupational Therapy

1051   *American Occupational Therapy Association Inc.*, 1383 Piccard Drive, Rockville, MD 20850, USA.

1052 *Australian Association of Occupational Therapists*, 17 Anchorage Street, St Clair, New South Wales 2759, Australia.

1053 *British Association of Occupational Therapists*, 6/8 Marshalsea Road, London SE1 1HL, England.

1054 *British Society of Hand Therapists*, (Mrs M. Ellis), Occupational Therapy Department, The London Hospital, Whitechapel Road, London E1 1BB, England.
Meetings offer an opportunity to present both clinical and research papers related to work with hand injuries.

1055 *Canadian Association of Occupational Therapists*, 3rd Floor, 110 Eglinton Avenue West, Toronto, Ontario, Canada M4R 1A3.

1056 *College of Occupational Therapists*, 6/8 Marshalsea Road, London SE1 1HL, England.
Special-interest groups associated with the College of Occupational Therapists: contacts and addresses change, but are regularly updated in the *British Journal of Occupational Therapy* [311].

1056a Alcohol and Substance Misuse, (Mrs B. Narang), Alcohol and Drug Units, Bexley Hospital, Old Bexley Lane, Bexley, Kent DA5 2BW, England.

1056b Care of the Elderly, (Ms P. Wheeler), Wonford House Hospital, Dryden Road, Wonford, Exeter, Devon EX2 5AF, England.

1056c Community Occupational Therapy in Mental Health, (Mrs R. Middlemiss), Mental Health Department, East Birmingham Hospital, Yardley Green Unit, Yardley Green Road, Birmingham B9 5PX, England.

1056d Development and Research in Psychiatry, (Mrs N. Bennie), Occupational Therapy Department, Gartnavel Royal Hospital, 1055 Great Western Road, Glasgow G12 0XH, Scotland.

1056e Mental Handicap, (Ms R. Bond), Occupational Therapy Department, St Ann's Hospital, Haven Road, Canford Cliffs, Poole, Dorset BH13 7LN, England.

1056f Mental Health, (Ms C. Greensmith), Occupational Therapy Department, The London Hospital, Whitechapel Road, London E1 1BB, England.

1056g Microcomputers, (Mrs C. V. MacCaul), Occupational Therapy Department, Christchurch College, North Holmes Road, Canterbury, Kent CT1 1QU, England.

1056h Neurology, (Ms J. Durkin), Occupational Therapy Department, Regional Neurological Rehabilitation Unit, Homerton Hospital, Homerton Row, London E9 6SR, England.

1056i Orthotics and Prosthetics, (Mrs R. Cooper), Occupational Therapy Department, Pinderfields General Hospital, Aberford Road, Wakefield, West Yorkshire WF1 4DG, England.

1056j Paediatrics, (Mrs K. Jasinska), Priory Care Unit, Priory Manor Child Development Centre, 1 Blagdon Road, London SE13, England.

1056k Perception, (Mrs G. Allan), 11 Buchanan Gardens, Hamilton Road, Mount Vernon, Glasgow G32 9QY, Scotland.

1056l Remedial Gardening, (Mr J. Catlin), Occupational Therapy Department, Psychiatric Unit, Chase Farm Hospital, The Ridgeway, Enfield, Middlesex EN2 8JL, England.

1056m Rheumatology, (Miss G. Rowbotham), Rheumatology Unit, Nuffield Orthopaedic Centre, Headington, Oxford OX3 7LD, England.

1057 *Interact*, (Mr W. E. Scott), Dept of Postgraduate Medical Education, University of Glasgow, Glasgow G12 8QQ, Scotland.

1058 *Scottish Society of Rehabilitation Medicine*, (Dr E. Cay), Rehabilitation Medicine Unit, University of Edinburgh, Astley Ainslie Hospital, Grange Loan, Edinburgh EH9 2HL, Scotland.

1059 *Society for Research in Rehabilitation*, (Mr P. Cornes), Rehabilitation Studies Unit, University of Edinburgh, 3 Lauriston Park, Edinburgh EH3 9JA, Scotland.
Founded in 1978 by a small group of doctors who thought there was a need to promote a scientific approach to the study of medical rehabilitation; abstracts of the proceedings of twice-yearly wide-ranging meetings were published in *International Journal of Rehabilitation Research* [45] and are now in *Clinical Rehabilitation* [41] for a trial period.

Physiotherapy

1060 *American Academy of Physical Medicine and Rehabilitation*, 122 South Michigan Avenue, Chicago, IL 60603, USA.

1061 *American Physical Therapy Association*, 1111 North Fairfax Street, Alexandria, VA 22314, USA.

1062 *Association des Kinésithérapeutes de Belgique (AKB)*, Grote Markt 26, 8970 Poperinge, Belgium.

1063 *Australian Physiotherapy Association*, 141 St George's Road, North Fitzroy, Victoria 3068, Australia.

1064 *Canadian Physiotherapy Association*, Suite 201, 44 Eglinton Avenue West, Toronto, Ontario, Canada.

1065 *Chartered Society of Physiotherapy (CSP)*, 14 Bedford Row, London WC1R 4ED, England.

1066 *Danske Fusioterapeuter (DF)*, Norre Voldgade 90, 1358 København K, Denmark.

1067 *Fédération Française des Masseurs Kinésithérapeutes Rééducateurs (FFMKR)*, 9/11 Rue des Petits Hôtels, 75010 Paris, France.

1068 *Gesellschaft für Physiotherapie der DDR*, Hainstrasse 17, 7010 Leipzig, GDR.

1069 *Kneippärztebund eV – Ärztlicher Gesellschaft für Physiotherapie (KAB)*, 8939 Bad Worishofen, Postfach 475, FRG.

1070 *Legitmerade Sjukgymnasters Riksforbund*, Apelbergsgatan 50, 111 37 Stockholm, Sweden.

1071 *Nederlands Genootschap voor Fysioterapie*, Postbus 248, Van Hogendorplaan 8, 3800 AE Amersfoort, Netherlands.

1072 *Norske Fysioterapeuters Fobund (NFF)*, Motzfeldtsgate 3, Oslo 1, Norway.

1073 *Schweizerischer Verband Staatlich Anerkannter Physiotherapeuten (SVP)*, Postfach 516, 8027 Zürich, Switzerland.

1074 *South African Society of Physiotherapy*, PO Box 47238, Parklands, Johannesburg 2121, South Africa.

1075 *Suomen Laakintavoimistelijaliito (SL)*, Asemamiehenkatu 4, 00520 Helsinki 52, Finland.

1076 *Turkiye Fizikoterapi ve Rehabiliasyon Cemiyeti Fizikoterapi Klinigi*, Capa, Istanbul, Turkey.

1077 *United States Physical Therapy Association*, 1803 Avon Lane, Arlington Heights, IL 60004, USA.

1078   *Vlaams Kinesitherapueten Verbond (VKV)*, Boeschepestraat 70, 8970 Poperinge, Belgium.

Dietetics, Nutrition

1079   *American Dietetic Association*, Suite 1100, 208 LaSalle Street, Chicago, IL 60604–1003, USA.

1080   *Association of French-speaking Dieticians*, 17 Rue Henri Bocquillon, 75013 Paris, France.

1081   *British Dietetic Association*, 7th floor, Elizabeth House, Suffolk Street, Birmingham B1 1LS, England.

1082   *Canadian Dietetic Association*, Suite 604, 480 University Avenue, Toronto, Ontario, Canada M5G 1V2.

1083   *Deutsche Gesellschaft für Ernährung*, Feldbergstrasse 28, Frankfurt am Main 6000, FRG.

1084   *Gesellschaft für Ernährung DDR*, (Dr W. Rodel), 1505 Bergholz, Rehbrucke-am-Luchgraben 7, GDR.

1085   *Hospital Caterers' Association*, 43 Royston Road, Penge, London SE20 7QW, England.

1086   *Nutrition Society*, Grosvenor Gardens House, 35–37 Grosvenor Gardens, London SW1W 0BS, England.

1087   *South African Dietetics Association*, Department of Home Economics, University of Stellenbosch, Stellenbosch 7600, South Africa.

Speech Therapy

1088   *American Speech–Language–Hearing Association (ASHA)*, 10801 Rockville Pike, Rockville, MD 20852, USA.

1089   *Australian Association of Speech and Hearing*, 212 Clarendon Terrace, East Melbourne, Victoria 3002, Australia.

1090   *British Association of Teachers of the Deaf*, (Secretary, Miss S. Dowe), Service for the Hearing Impaired, Icknield High School, Riddy Lane, Luton, Bedfordshire LU3 2AH, England.

1091   *Canadian Association of Speech–Language Pathologists and Audiologists*, Suite 1215, 25 Main Street West, Hamilton, Ontario, Canada L8P 1H1.

1092   *College of Speech Therapists*, Harold Poster House, 6 Lechmere Road, London NW2 5BU, England.

1093   *Linguistics Association of Great Britain*, (Secretary, Dr R. Coates), School of Cognitive and Computing Sciences, University of Sussex, Falmer, Brighton BN1 9QN, England.

1094   *National Association of Professionals Concerned with Language Impaired Children* (*NAPLIC*), 93 Chestnut Copse, Hurst Green, Oxted, Surrey RH8 0JJ, England.

1095   *New Zealand Speech–Language Therapists' Association*, PO Box 38–117, Petone, Wellington, New Zealand.

1096   *South African Speech and Hearing Association*, PO Box 31782, Braamfontein 2017, South Africa.

Radiography

1097   *American Society of Radiologic Technologists*, Suite 1820, 55 E. Jackson Boulevard, Chicago, IL 60604, USA.

1098   *Asociación Española de Técnicos en Radiología*, Conde de Penalvar 92, 28006 Madrid, Spain.

1099   *Association Française du Personnel Paramédical d'Electroradiologie*, Boîte Postale 9, Cedex 13, 75634 Paris, France.

1100   *Australian Institute of Radiography*, PO Box 278, East Melbourne, Victoria 3002, Australia.

1101   *British Institute of Radiology*, 36 Portland Place, London W1N 4AT, England.

1102   *Canadian Association of Medical Radiation Technologists*, Suite 410, 280 Metcalfe Street, Ottawa, Ontario, Canada K2P 1R7.

1103   *College of Radiographers*, 14 Upper Wimpole Street, London W1M 8BN, England.

1104   *Czechoslovak Society of Radiological Technicians*, (Mr V. L. Jarkovsky), University Hospital, Marxova 13, Pilza, Czechoslovakia.

1105   *Deutscher Verein für Technische Assistenten in Medizin*, Holsterhauser Strasse 69, Essen 43, FRG.

1106   *Japanese Association of Radiologic Technologists*, 1–26–7 Shinkawa, Chuo-Ku, Tokyo 104, Japan.

1107   *Medical Radiological Technicians of Belgium*, Boîte Postale 112, 4000 Liège, Belgium.

1108   *Nederlands Vereniging van Radiologisch Laboranten*, Catharijnesigel 73, 3511 GM Utrecht, Netherlands.

1109   *Norsk Radiograffarbund*, Post Box 9202, Vaterland 0134, Oslo 1, Norway.

1110   *Royal College of Radiologists*, 38 Portland Place, London W1N 4AT, England.

1111   *Schweizerisch Vereinigung für Medizinische-Technische Radiologie-assistenten*, PO Box 4011, Basel, Switzerland.

1112   *Singapore Society of Radiographers*, Singapore Professional Centre, 2nd Floor, Block 23, Outram Park, Singapore 0310.

1113   *Society of Radiographers*, 14 Upper Wimpole Street, London W1M 8BN, England.

1114   *Society of Radiographers of Jamaica*, PO Box 38, Kingston 6, Jamaica.

1115   *Suomen Rontgenhoitajat RY* (Society of Radiographers in Finland), Asemamiehenhatu 4, 00520 Helsinki, Finland.

1116   *Verband der Diplomierten Radiologisch-technischen Assistentinnen und Assistenten Österreichs*, Simmeringer, Haupstrasse 34/1/IVI, 1110 Wien, Austria.

1117   *Verein für Medizinische, Technische und Radiologische Assistenten*, Strahlenklinik, Voss Strasse 3, Heidelberg 69, FRG.

Other Health Care and Rehabilitation

1118   *American Association for Rehabilitation Therapy*, Box 93, North Little Rock, AR 72116, USA.

1119   *American Corrective Therapy Association*, 259-08 148 Road, Rosedale, NY 11422, USA.

1120   *American Dance Therapy Association*, 2000 Century Plaza, Suite 230, Columbia, MD 21044, USA.

1121   *British Association of Art Therapists Ltd*, 13C Northwood Road, Highgate, London N6 5TL, England.

1122   *British Association for Drama Therapists*, PO Box 98, Kirkbymoorside, North Yorkshire YO6 6EX, England.

1123   *British Society for Music Therapy*, Guildhall School of Music and Drama, Barbican, London EC2Y 8DT, England.

3   ASSOCIATIONS, INSTITUTIONS, ORGANIZATIONS

Further lists of relevant associations and societies can be found in Zeitak and Berman [168], Henderson and Henderson [160], and Darnbrough and Kinrade [153]; and in information published by the Disabled Living Foundation [156] and Disability Scotland [325].

Chiropody

Institutions offering training in chiropody are listed in Alexander's *Directory of schools of medicine . . .*, pp. 529–30, 555–6, 562–4 [199].

1124   *British Footwear Manufacturers' Federation*, Royalty House, 72 Dean Street, London W1, England.

1125   *Foot Health Council*, 84–88 Great Eastern Street, London EC2A 3ED, England.
Footwear Advisory Service, *Disabled Living Foundation* [1241].

1126   *Langer Biomechanics Group (UK)*, The Green, Cheadle, Stoke-on-Trent ST10 1RL, England.

1127   *London Postgraduate Study Group*, 13a Stuart Crescent, Wood Green, London N22 5NJ, England.

1128   *Shoe and Allied Trades Research Association, SATRA*, Satra House, Rockingham Road, Kettering, Northamptonshire NN16 9JH, England.

Occupational Therapy

Institutions offering training in occupational therapy (either graduate or postgraduate) are listed in Alexander's *Directory of schools of medicine . . .*, pp. 534, 545–7 [199].

British Institute of Mental Handicap [1235].

1129   *Centre on Environment for the Handicapped*, 35 Great Smith Street, London SW1P 3BJ, England. (From 1990, Centre on Accessible Environments.)

1130   *DIAL UK*, Victoria Buildings, 117 High Street, Clay Cross, Chesterfield, Derbyshire S45 9DZ, England.

1131   *Disability Alliance*, 25 Denmark Street, London WC2H 8NJ, England.

Disabled Living Foundation [1241]

1132   *Royal Association for Disability and Rehabilitation, RADAR*, 25 Mortimer Street, London W1N 8AB, England.

Physiotherapy

Institutions offering training in physiotherapy are listed in Alexander's *Directory of schools of medicine . . .*, pp. 536, 542–5, [199].

1133   *British Association of Sport and Medicine*, 39 Linkfield Road, Mountsorrel, near Loughborough, Leicestershire LE12 7DJ, England.

1134   *British Sports Association for the Disabled*, Hayward House, Barnard Crescent, Aylesbury, Buckinghamshire HP21 9PP, England.

1135   *London Institute of Sports Medicine*, c/o St Bartholomew's Hospital Medical College, Charterhouse Square, London EC1M 6BQ, England.
Publishes *Sports Medicine Bulletin* [229]

1136   *Schweizerischer Verband für Behindertensport*, Bürglistrasse 11, 8002 Zürich, Switzerland.

Dietetics, Nutrition

Institutions offering training in dietetics and nutrition (either graduate or postgraduate) are listed in Alexander's *Directory of schools of medicine . . .*, pp. 531, 539–40 [199].

1137   *British Nutrition Foundation*, 15 Belgrave Square, London SW1X 8PS, England.

1138   *Coeliac Society*, PO Box 220, High Wycombe, Buckinghamshire HP11 2HY, England.

1139   *Colostomy Welfare Group*, 39 Eccleston Square, London SW1V 1PB, England.

1140 *Familial Hypercholinesterolaemia Association*, PO Box 133, High Wycombe, Buckinghamshire HP13 6LF, England.

1141 *Food and Drink Federation*, 6 Catherine Street, London WC2B 5JJ, England.

1142 *Food Research Association*, Randalls Road, Leatherhead, Surrey KT22 7RY, England.

1143 *London Food Commission*, 88 Old Street, London EC1 9AR, England.

Market Information Service, *Food Research Association* [1142].

1144 *National Dairy Council*, 7 John Princes Street, London W1M 0AP, England.

1145 *Oxford Nutrition*, PO Box 31, Oxford OX2 6HB, England.

1146 *Vegan Society Ltd*, 47 Highlands Road, Leatherhead, Surrey KT22 8NQ, England.

Speech Therapy

Institutions offering training in speech therapy are listed in Alexander's *Directory of schools of medicine . . .*, pp. 600, 605 [199].

Note: There are equivalent organizations to several of these English associations in Scotland, Wales and Northern Ireland; in the interests of brevity these have been omitted.

1147 *Action for Dysphasic Adults*, 37A Royal Street, Lambeth, London SE1 7LL, England.

1148 *Aid for Children with Tracheostomies*, c/o Secretary, Station House, Station Road, Market Bosworth, Nuneaton, Warwickshire CV13 0PE, England.

1149 *Association For All Speech Impaired Children (AFASIC)* 347 Central Markets, Smithfield, London EC1A 9NH, England.

1150 *Association for Stammerers*, c/o Finsbury Centre, Pine Street, London EC1R 0JH, England.

1151 *Blissymbolics Communications Resource Centre*, Thomas House, South Glamorgan Institute of Higher Education, Cyncoed Centre, Cyncoed Road, Cardiff CF2 6XD, Wales.

1152 *British Aphasiology Society*, (Ms Rachel David), School of Speech Therapy, City of Birmingham Polytechnic, Franchise Street, Perry Barr, Birmingham B42 2SU, England.

1153 *British Association of the Hard of Hearing, BAHOH*, 7/11 Armstrong Road, London W3 7JL, England.

1154 *British Deaf Association*, 38 Victoria Place, Carlisle CA1 1HU, England.

1155 *Cleft Lip and Palate Association*, 1 Eastwood Gardens, Kenton, Newcastle upon Tyne NE3 3DQ, England.

1156 *International Society for Augmentative and Alternative Communication*, PO Box 1762, Station R, Toronto, Ontario, Canada M4G 4A3, and c/o *RADAR* [1132].

1157 *Makaton Vocabulary Development Project*, 31 Firwood Drive, Camberley, Surrey, England.

1158 *National Association of Laryngectomee Clubs*, 39 Eccleston Square, London SW1V 1PB, England.

1159 *National Centre for Cued Speech*, 29–30 Watling Street, Canterbury, Kent CT1 2UD, England.

1160 *National Deaf Children's Society*, 45 Hereford Road, London W2 5AH, England.

1161 *National Deaf-Blind and Rubella Association, SENSE*, 311 Gray's Inn Road, London WC1X 8PT, England.

1162 *Paget Gorman Society*, (Development Officer, Bob Newey), 3 Gipsy Lane, Headington, Oxford OX3 7PT, England.

1163 *Royal Association in Aid of the Deaf and Dumb*, 27 Old Oak Road, Acton, London W3 7HN, England.

Royal National Institute for the Deaf (RNID) [1262].

1164 *Speech Foundation of America*, PO Box 11749, Memphis, TN 38111, USA.

1165 *Voice Research Society*, 59 Southbrook Road, Lee, London SE12 8LJ, England.

1166   *Voluntary Organizations Communication and Language* (*VOCAL*), 336 Brixton Road, London SW9 7AA, England.

Radiography

Institutions offering training in radiography are listed in Alexander's *Directory of schools of medicine . . .*, pp. 537, 547–554 [199].

1167   *Breast Care and Mastectomy Association* (*BCMA*), 26a Harrison Street, King's Cross, London WC1H 8JG, England, and 9 Castle Terrace, Edinburgh EH1 2DP, Scotland.

1168   *British Association of Cancer United Patients*, *BACUP*, 121/123 Charterhouse Street, London EC1M 3AA, England.

1169   *Cancer Aftercare and Rehabilitation Society, CARE*, 21 Zetland Road, Redland, Bristol BS6 7AH, England.

Cancer Education and Co-ordinating Group of the UK and Republic of Ireland, c/o Secretary, *Ulster Cancer Foundation* [1181].

1170   *Cancer Link*, 46A Pentonville Road, London N1 9HF, England, and 9 Castle Terrace, Edinburgh EH1 2DP, Scotland.

1171   *Cancer Relief Macmillan Fund*, Anchor House, 15/19 Britten Street, London SW3 3TZ, England, and 9 Castle Terrace, Edinburgh EH1 2DP, Scotland.

1172   *Cancer Research Campaign* (*CRC*), 2 Carlton House Terrace, London W1Y 5AR, England.

1173   *Cancer Research Campaign, Education and Child Studies Research Group*, University of Manchester, Kinnaird Road, Manchester M20 9QL, England.

1174   *Hodgkin's Disease Association*, PO Box 275, Haddenham, Aylesbury, Buckinghamshire HP17 8JJ, England.

1175   *Irish Cancer Society*, 5 Northumberland Road, Dublin 4, Eire.

1176   *Leukaemia Research Fund*, 43 Great Ormond Street, London WC1N 3JJ, England.

1177   *Leukaemia Care Society*, PO Box 82, Exeter, Devon EX2 5DP, England.

1178   *Malcolm Sargent Cancer Fund for Children*, 14 Abingdon Road, London W8 6AF, England.

1179   *Marie Curie Cancer Care*, 28 Belgrave Square, London SW1X 8QG, England.

1180   *South West Thames Regional Cancer Organisation*, Block E, Royal Marsden Hospital, Downs Road, Sutton, Surrey SM2 5PT, England.
Other British Regional Health Authorities have similar Regional Cancer Organizations, such as [1182].

1181   *Ulster Cancer Foundation*, 40/42 Eglantine Avenue, Belfast BT9 6DX, Northern Ireland.

1182   *Wessex Regional Cancer Organization*, Royal South Hants Hospital, Graham Road, Southampton SO9 4PE, England.

1183   *Women's National Cancer Control Campaign*, 1 South Audley Street, London W1Y 5DQ, England.

Other Health Care and Rehabilitation

Note: There are equivalent organizations to several of these English associations in Scotland, Wales and Northern Ireland; in the interests of brevity these have been omitted.

1184   *Action Against Allergy*, 43 The Downs, London SW20 8HS, England.

1185   *Action for Research into Multiple Sclerosis (ARMS)*, 11 Dartmouth Street, London SW1, England. *ARMS Research Unit*, Central Middlesex Hospital, Acton Lane, London NW10 7NS, England.

1186   *American Association on Mental Retardation*, 5201 Connecticut Avenue NW, Washington, DC 20015, USA.

1187   *Anorexic Aid*, Priory Centre, 11 Priory Road, High Wycombe, Buckinghamshire HP13 6SL, England.

ARMS, *Action for Research into Multiple Sclerosis* [1185].

1188   *Arthritis and Rheumatism Council*, 41 Eagle Street, London WC1R 4AR, England.

1189   *Association to Aid the Sexual and Personal Relationships of People with a Disability (SPOD)*, 286 Camden Road, London N7 0BJ, England.

1190   *British Colostomy Association*, 38/39 Eccleston Square, London SW1V 1PB, England.

1191   *British Diabetic Association*, 10 Queen Anne Street, London W1M 0BD, England.

British Institute of Mental Handicap [1235].

1192   *British Kidney Patients' Association*, Bordon, Hampshire GU35 9JS, England.

1193   *British Rheumatism and Arthritis Association*, 6 Grosvenor Crescent, London SW1X 7ER, England.

1194   *Canadian Rehabilitation Council for the Disabled*, Suite 2110, One Yonge Street, Toronto, Ontario, Canada M5E 1E5.

1195   *Coronary Prevention Group*, Central Middlesex Hospital, Acton Lane, London NW10 7NS, England.

1196   *Council for Exceptional Children*, 1920 Association Drive, Reston, Arlington, VA 22091, USA.

1197   *Cystic Fibrosis Research Trust*, Alexander House, 5 Blyth Road, Bromley, Kent BR1 3RS, England.

1198   *Disabilities Studies Unit*, Wildhanger, Amberley, Arundel, West Sussex BN18 9NR, England.

Disabled Living Foundation [1241].

1199   *Down's Syndrome Association*, 12/13 Clapham Common Southside, London SW4 7AA, England.

1200   *Foresight*, The Old Vicarage, Witley, Godalming, Surrey GU8 5PN, England.

1201   *Friedrich's Ataxia Group*, Burleigh Lodge, Knowle Lane, Cranleigh, Surrey GU6 8RD, England.

1202   *Handikappininstitutet*, Box 303, 161 26 Bromma, Sweden.

1203   *Headway, National Head Injuries Association*, 200 Mansfield Road, Nottingham NG1 3HX, England.

1204   *Invalid Children's Aid Nationwide*, Allen Graham House, 198 City Road, London EC1V 2PH, England.

MENCAP, Royal Society for Mentally Handicapped Children and Adults [1217].

MIND, *National Association for Mental Health* [1209].

1205 *Motor Neurone Disease Association*, 61 Derngate, Northampton, North-amptonshire NN1 1UE, England

1206 *Multiple Sclerosis Society*, 286 Munster Road, Fulham, London SW6 6AP, England.

1207 *Muscular Dystrophy Society*, Natrass House, 35 Macaulay Road, London SW4 0QP, England.

1208 *National Association for Colitis and Crohn's Disease*, 98a London Road, St Albans, Hertfordshire AL1 1NX, England.

1209 *National Association for Mental Health* (*MIND*), 22 Harley Street, London W1N 2ED, England.

1210 *National Association for the Welfare of Children in Hospital* (*NAWCH*), Argyle House, 29–31 Euston Road, London NW1, England.

1211 *National Autistic Society*, 276 Willesden Lane, London NW2 5RB, England.

1212 *National Bureau for Handicapped Students*, 40 Brunswick Square, London WC1, England.

1213 *National Council for Special Education*, 1 Wood Street, Stratford-upon-Avon, Warwickshire CV37 6JE, England.

National Head Injuries Association, Headway [1203].

1214 *National Rehabilitation Association*, 633 S. Washington Street, Alexandria, VA 22314, USA.

1215 *National Society for Phenylketonuria and Allied Disorders*, 14 Newfoundland Drive, Cringleford, Norwich, Norfolk, England.

Northern Ireland Council on Disability [1257].

1216 *Prader Willi Syndrome Association*, 30 Follett Drive, Abbot's Langley, Hertfordshire WD5 0LP, England.

1217 *Royal Society for Mentally Handicapped Children and Adults, MENCAP*, 117–123 Golden Lane, London EC1Y 0RT, England.

1218   *Schizophrenia Association of Great Britain*, International Schizophrenia Centre, Bryn Hyfryd, The Crescent, Bangor, Gwynedd LL57 2AG, Wales.

1219   *Scottish Council on Disability*, Princes House, 5 Shandwick Place, Edinburgh EH2 4RG, Scotland. (From 1990, *Disability Scotland*.)

1220   *Spastics Society*, 12 Park Crescent, London W1N 4EQ, England.

SPOD, Association to Aid the Sexual and Personal Relationships of People with a Disability [1189].

4   GOVERNMENT BODIES

International

1221   *World Health Organization*, 20 Avenue Appia, 1211 Geneva 27, Switzerland.

European Community

1222   *EC Commission*, 8 Storey's Gate, London SW1P 3AT, England.

United Kingdom

Chiropodists Board, Council for Professions Supplementary to Medicine [1223].

1223   *Council for Professions Supplementary to Medicine (CPSM)*, Park House, 184 Kennington Park Road, London SE11 4BU, England.

Dietitians' Board, Council for Professions Supplementary to Medicine [1223].

1224   *Data Protection Registrar*, Springfield House, Water Lane, Wilmslow, Cheshire SK9 5AY, England.

1225   *Department of Agriculture and Fisheries in Scotland*, Chesser House, 500 Gorgie Road, Edinburgh EH11 3AW, Scotland.

1226   *Department of Education and Science*, Elizabeth House, York Road, London SE1 7PH, England.

1227   *Department of Health*, Hannibal House, Elephant and Castle, London SE1 6TE, England.

1228   *Dietetic Officer, Department of Health*, Hannibal House, Elephant and Castle, London SE1 6TE, England.

1229   *Health and Safety Executive*, (Public Enquiry Point), Room 414, St Hugh's House, Stanley Precinct, Bootle, Merseyside L20 3QY, England.

1230   *Health Education Authority (HEA)*, Hamilton House, Mabledon Place, London WC1H 9TX, England.

1231   *Ministry of Agriculture, Fisheries and Food (MAFF)*, Horseferry Road, London SW1P 2AE, England.

Occupational Therapists Board, Council for Professions Supplementary to Medicine [1223].

1232   *Office of Population Censuses and Surveys*, St Catherine's House, 10 Kingsway, London WC2B 6JP, England.

Physiotherapists Board, Council for Professions Supplementary to Medicine [1223].

Radiographers Board, Council for Professions Supplementary to Medicine [1223].

1233   *Scottish Home and Health Department, SHHD*, St Andrew's House, Edinburgh EH1 3DE, Scotland.

United States of America

1234   *Rehabilitation Services Administration*, Mary E. Switzer Building, Room 3212, 330 C Street SW, Washington, DC 20202, USA.

5   LIBRARIES, INFORMATION CENTRES AND MUSEUMS

United Kingdom

1235   *British Institute of Mental Handicap*, Wolverhampton Road, Kidderminster, Worcestershire DY10 3PP, England.

1236   *British Library Document Supply Centre*, Boston Spa, Wetherby, West Yorkshire LS23 7BQ, England.

1237   *British Library Humanities and Social Sciences*, Great Russell Street, London WC1B 3DG, England.

British Library Medical Information Service, British Library DSC [1236].

1238   *British Library Science Reference and Information Service*, 25 Southampton Buildings, Chancery Lane, London WC2A 1AW, England.

1239 *British Medical Association*, Nuffield Library, BMA House, Tavistock Square, London WC1H 9JP, England.

C. and J. Clark, Street Shoe Museum [1269].

1240 *Department of Health Library*, Hannibal House, Elephant and Castle, London SE1 6TE, England.

1241 *Disabled Living Foundation*, 380 Harrow Road, London W9 2HU, England. A list of disabled living centres in England is found in *British Medical Journal*, 1988, **296**, 1053.

1242 *East Anglian Regional Health Authority libraries*, (RLG representative, Mr Peter Morgan), Cambridge University Medical Library, Addenbrooke's Hospital, Hills Road, Cambridge CB2 2QQ, England.

1243 *Footman Collection*, on display at the Old Post Office Savings Bank, Grove Mill, Mitcham, Surrey, England.
Appointments to view may be made by contacting Miss D. Whitwam at the Science Museum, South Kensington, London SW7 2DD, England, telephone 071-938 8070. (This is a temporary arrangement while the contents are researched and catalogued before removal to the Science Museum, probably in 1991.)

Health and Safety Executive [1229].

Health Education Authority (HEA) [1230].

Health Search Scotland, Scottish Health Education Group [1264].

1244 *Help for Health*, Patient Care Information Service, Wessex Region Library Unit, South Academic Block, Southampton General Hospital, Southampton SO9 4XY, England.

1245 *Hospice Information Service*, St Christopher's Hospice, 51/59 Lawrie Park Road, Sydenham, London SE26 6DZ, England.

1246 *Institute of Laryngology and Otology*, Royal National Throat Nose and Ear Hospital, 330/332 Gray's Inn Road, London WC1X 8EE, England.

1247 *Institute of Neurology*, Rockefeller Medical Library, National Hospitals for Nervous Diseases, Queen Square, London WC1N 3BG, England.

1248 *Institute of Orthopaedics*, Royal National Orthopaedic Hospital, Bolsover Street, London W1N 6AD, England.

1249   *King's Fund Centre*, 126 Albert Street, London NW1 7NF, England.
This extensive reference library can be used by anyone interested in the health services, and there is an information service for those who are unable to visit.

1250   *Library Association*, 7 Ridgmount Street, London WC1E 7HR, England. The *Medical, Health and Welfare Libraries Group* and *Nursing Information SubGroup* can be contacted at the same address.

1251   *Merseyside Regional Health Authority libraries*, (RLG representative, Mr Derrick Crook), Librarian, Liverpool Medical Institution, 114 Mount Pleasant, Liverpool L3 5SR, England.

1252   *National Hospitals College of Speech Sciences*, Chandler House, 2 Wakefield Street, London WC1N 1PG, England.

National Hospitals for Nervous Diseases, Institute of Neurology [1247].

1253   *North East Thames Regional Library Service*, David Ferriman Library, North Middlesex Hospital, Sterling Way, London N18 1QX, England.
Directory of libraries and information services within the Region is available.

1254   *North West Thames Regional Library Service*, c/o Westminster Site Library, Charing Cross & Westminster Medical School, 17 Horseferry Road, London SW1P 2AR, England.

1255   *North Western Regional Health Authority libraries*, (RLG representative, Ms Anne Strange, District Librarian), Royal Preston Hospital, Sharoe Green Lane, Fulwood, Preston PR2 4HT, England.

1256   *Northampton Central Museum and Art Gallery*, Guildhall Road, Northampton, Northamptonshire NN1 1DP, England.

1257   *Northern Ireland Council on Disability*, Information Service for Disabled People, 2 Annandale Avenue, Belfast BT7 3JR, Northern Ireland.

1258   *Northern Ireland Health & Social Services Library Queen's University Medical Library*, Institute of Clinical Science, Grosvenor Road, Belfast BT12 6BJ, Northern Ireland.

1259   *Northern Regional Health Authority libraries*, (RLG representative, Mrs Kath O'Donovan), University Medical and Dental Library, The Medical School, Framlington Place, Newcastle upon Tyne NE2 4HH, England.

1260   *Nuffield Centre for Health Service Studies*, Clarendon Road, Leeds LS2 9PL, England.

Office of Population Censuses and Surveys, Information Branch [1232].

1261   *Oxford Regional Library & Information Service*, Cairns Library, John Radcliffe Hospital, Headington, Oxford OX3 9DU, England.

1262   *Royal National Institute for the Deaf, RNID*, 105 Gower Street, London WC1E 6AH, England.

Royal National Throat Nose and Ear Hospital, Institute of Laryngology and Otology [1246].

1263   *Royal Society of Medicine*, 1 Wimpole Street, London W1M 8AE, England.

1264   *Scottish Health Education Group*, Woodburn House, Canaan Lane, Edinburgh EH10 4SG, Scotland.

1265   *Scottish Health Service Centre*, Crewe Road South, Edinburgh EH4 2LF, Scotland.

1266   *South East Thames Regional Library Service*, SE Thames Regional Health Authority, Thrift House, Collington Avenue, Bexhill-on-Sea, East Sussex, England.

1267   *South West Thames Regional Library Service*, Royal Surrey County Hospital, Guildford, Surrey GU2 5XX, England.

1268   *South Western Regional Health Authority libraries*, (RLG representative, Mrs Pam Prior, Librarian), Medical Library, Torbay Hospital, Torquay, Devon TQ2 7AA, England.

1269   *Street Shoe Museum* (C. and J. Clark), Street, Somerset BA16 0YA, England.

1270   *Trent Regional Health Authority libraries*, (RLG representative, Mr Graham Matthews), Staff Library, Rotherham District Hospital, Moorgate Road, Rotherham, South Yorkshire S60 2UD, England.

1271   *Wales*, (RLG representative, Mr John Lancaster), Main Library, University of Wales College of Medicine, University Hospital of Wales, Heath Park, Cardiff CF4 4XN, Wales.

1272   *Welsh Health Promotion Authority*, Heron House, 35/43 Newport Road, Cardiff CF2 1SB, Wales.

1273   *West Midlands Regional Health Authority libraries*, (RLG representative, Mrs Janet Claridge, Medical Sub-Librarian), Barnes Library, Medical School, University of Birmingham, Vincent Drive, Birmingham B15 2TJ, England.

1274   *Wessex Regional Library Information Service*, South Academic Block, Southampton General Hospital, Southampton SO9 4XY, England.

1275   *Wessex Regional Orthopaedic Centre*, Lord Mayor Treloar Hospital, Alton, Hampshire GU34 1RJ, England.

1276   *Whitefield Centre*, Special Needs Library and Information Service, Macdonald Road, Walthamstow, London E17 4AZ, England.

1277   *Yorkshire Regional Health Authority Libraries*, (RLG representative, Mr Ian King, District Librarian), Bradford Royal Infirmary, Duckford Lane, Duckford, Bradford, West Yorkshire BD9 6RJ, England.

United States of America

1278   *American Library Association*, 50 East Huron Street, Chicago, IL 60611, USA.

1279   *Center for the History of Footcare and Footwear*, Pennsylvania College of Podiatric Medicine, Eight at Race Street, Philadelphia, PA 19107, USA.

1280   *Medical Library Association*, Suite 300, 6 North Michigan Avenue, Chicago, IL 60602, USA.

1281   *National Library of Medicine*, 8600 Rockville Pike, Rockville, Bethesda, MD 20209, USA.

6 SELECTED PUBLISHERS AND BOOKSELLERS

This list is necessarily very selective, since publishers' addresses can be found from a variety of sources. *Whitaker's Books in Print* [102] and *Books in Print* [103] both list British and foreign publishers and their addresses; the following also include lists of publishers:

1282   **Cassell** and the **Publishers Association**. *Directory of Publishing*. London: Cassell. Annual.

1283   Curzon, M., ed. (1987). *5001 hard-to-find publishers and their addresses*. 3rd ed. London: Alan Armstrong.
Lists over 7500 publishers 'who produce books in English of UK or international interest'.

1284   *International Literary Market Place*. New York: Bowker. Published in alternate years.

1285   *LMP: Literary Market Place, the directory of American book publishing, with names and numbers*. New York: Bowker. Annual.

Many of the organizations mentioned above also publish material relevant to allied health: their addresses are not repeated here.

1286   *Alpha Academic*, Halfpenny Furze, Mill Lane, Chalfont St Giles, Buckinghamshire HP8 4NR, England.

1287   *Asgard Publishing Co.*, 4A The Square, Petersfield, Hampshire GU32 3HJ, England.

British Institute of Mental Handicap [1235].

1288   *British Library (Publication Sales Unit)*, Boston Spa, near Wetherby, West Yorkshire LS23 7BQ, England.

1289   *Carolando Press*, 6545 WN Avenue, Oak Park, Chicago, IL 60302, USA.

1290   *Chadwyck-Healey Ltd*, Cambridge Place, Cambridge CB2 1NR, England.

1291   *CINAHL Corporation*, PO Box 70572, East Pasadena, CA 91107–70572, USA.

1292   *Department of Education and Science, Publications Despatch Centre*, Government Buildings, Honeypot Lane, Stanmore, Middlesex HA7 1AZ, England.

1293   *DHSS Health Publications Unit*, No. 2 Site, Manchester Road, Heywood, Lancashire OL10 2PX, England.

1294   *DHSS (Leaflets)*, PO Box 21, Honeypot Lane, Stanmore, Middlesex HA7 1AY, England.

1295   *GJM Podiatry Books*, Oakgate Chambers, 20 Bath Place, Taunton, Somerset TA1 4ER, England.

Glendale Adventist Medical Center, now *CINAHL Corporation* [1291].

1296   *Helena Press*, Orchard Lane, Goathland, Whitby, North Yorkshire YO22 5JT, England.

1297   *Her Majesty's Stationery Office (HMSO)*, St Crispins, Duke Street, Norwich NR3 1PD, England.

1297a   HMSO Publications Centre (mail and telephone orders): PO Box 276, London SW8 5DT, England.

1297b   HMSO Bookshops: 49 High Holborn, London WC1V 6HB, England;
71 Lothian Road, Edinburgh EH3 9AZ, Scotland;
80 Chichester Street, Belfast BT1 4JY, Northern Ireland.

1298   *Kendall/Hunt Publishers*, 2460 Kerper Boulevard, Dubuque, IA 52001, USA.

1299   *Kingston Press Services*, 28 High Street, Teddington, Middlesex TW11 8EW, England.

1300   *Lanchester Library Publications*, Lanchester Polytechnic Library, Much Park Street, Coventry CV2 2HF, England.

1301   *Learning Development Aids*, Duke Street, Wisbech, Cambridgeshire PE13 2AE, England.

1302   *Majors Scientific Books*, 1851 Diplomat, Dallas, TX 75234, USA.

1303   *MIND Bookshop*, 4th floor, 24–32 Stephenson Way, London NW1 2HD, England.

1304   *Ministry of Agriculture, Fisheries and Food*, Lion House, Willowburn Estate, Alnwick, Northumberland NE66 2PF, England.

1305   *Multilingual Matters*, Bank House, 8A Hill Road, Clevedon, Avon BS21 7HH, England.

National Library of Medicine [1281].

1306   *NFER-Nelson Publishing Co. Ltd*, Darville House, 2 Oxford Road East, Windsor, Berkshire SL4 1DF, England.

1307   *Open University Educational Enterprises Ltd*, 12 Coffer Close, Stony Stratford, Milton Keynes, Northamptonshire MK11 1BY, England.

1308   *Rehabilitation International USA*, 20 West 40th Street, New York, NY 10018, USA.

1309   *Stanley Thornes (Publishers) Ltd*, Old Station Drive, Leckhampton, Cheltenham GL53 0DN, England.

1310   *University of Bradford, Food Policy Unit*, School of Biomedical Sciences, Richmond Road, Bradford, West Yorkshire BD7 1DP, England.

1311   *University of Manchester, Department of Community Medicine*, Oxford Road, Manchester M13 9PT, England.

1312   *Winslow Press*, Telford Road, Bicester, Oxfordshire OX6 0TS, England. Produce catalogues on *Occupational therapy* and *Rehabilitation materials for occupational therapy*, with a wide range of resources.

7 DATABASE PRODUCERS, HOSTS AND VENDORS

Ulrich's International periodicals directory [57], Vol. 3 contains a full list of *c.* 500 periodicals, abstracts and indexes that are available online, with a further section listing 40 hosts or vendors of a wide range of databases.

1313   *BARD* and *BARDSOFT*, British Database on Research into Aids for the Disabled, Handicapped Persons Research Unit, Newcastle upon Tyne Polytechnic, Coach Lane Campus, 1 Coach Lane, Newcastle upon Tyne NE7 7TW, England.

CINAHL Corporation [1291].

1314   *Data-Star*, Plaza Suite, 114 Jermyn Street, London SW1Y 6HJ, England. Database vendor.

DHSS-DATA, Department of Health Library [1240].

1315   *Dialog Information Services Inc.*, 3460 Hillview Avenue, Palo Alto, CA 94304, USA. Database vendor.

DLF-DATA, Disabled Living Foundation [1241].

1316   *EMBase*, Excerpta Medica, PO Box 1126, 1000 BC Amsterdam, Netherlands. Database producer

Healthbox, Help for Health [1244].

MEDLINE, National Library of Medicine [1281].

1317 *RECAL*, National Centre for Training and Education in Prosthetics and Orthotics, University of Strathclyde, Curran Building, 131 St James' Road, Glasgow G4 0LS, Scotland.

8 AUDIO-VISUAL AND NON-BOOK MATERIAL PRODUCERS

Many of the organizations mentioned above also publish material relevant to allied health: their addresses are not repeated here.

BMA/BLITHE Film and Video Library has ceased operation, but many of the medical and health films and videos are available from the *British Medical Association* Nuffield Library [1239].

1318 *Camera Talks*, 197 Botley Road, Oxford OX2 0HE, England.
Slide sets, 35 mm filmstrips, cassette tapes, 16 mm films.

1319 *Central Film Library*, PO Box 35, Wetherby, West Yorkshire LS23 7EX, England.
Films and videos on health education and special education: for sale and hire.

1320 *Concord Video and Film Council Ltd*, 201 Felixstowe Road, Ipswich, Suffolk IP3 9BJ, England.
Films and videos with emphasis on social issues; for hire. Catalogue of programmes on disability available.

1321 *CTVC Film and Video Library*, Beeson's Yard, Bury Lane, Rickmansworth, Hertfordshire WD3 IDS, England.

Disabled Living Foundation [1241] produces a list of distributors of audiovisual material on disability.

1322 *Graves Medical AudioVisual Library*, Holly House, 220 New London Road, Chelmsford, Essex CM2 9BJ, England.
Tape–slide programmes and videos, mainly of general medical interest; for sale and hire.

1323 *Guild Sound and Vision Ltd*, 6 Royce Road, Peterborough, Cambridgeshire PE1 5YB, England.
Health, social issues, medical; for sale and hire.

Health Education Authority (HEA) [1230].

1324 *Medical AudioVisual Information Service (MAVIS)*, Centre for Medical Education, Ninewells Hospital and Medical School, University of Dundee, Dundee DD1 9SY, Scotland.

Creates and maintains a national index of audio-visual materials on all medical and dental topics; provides an information retrieval service on such material.

1325   *Mental Health Film Council*, 22 Harley Street, London W1N 2ED, England.

1326   *National Audiovisual Aids Library*, Paxton Place, Gipsy Road, London SE27 9SR, England.
The catalogue of the Film Library for Teacher Education includes films and videos about special schools, children with cerebral palsy, mental subnormality, blindness and multiple handicaps.

1327   *Oxford Educational Resources Ltd*, 197 Botley Road, Oxford OX2 0HE, England.

1328   *Plymouth Medical Films*, 33 New Street, Barbican, Plymouth PL1 2NA, England.

1329   *Scottish Central Film Library*, Dowanhill, 74 Victoria Crescent Road, Glasgow G12 9JN, Scotland.
Films and videos on health education and special education; for sale and hire.

Scottish Health Education Group [1264].

1330   *Town and Country Productions*, 21 Cheyne Row, Chelsea, London SW3 5HP, England.
Includes documentary films on sports for disabled people, on the work of the Disabled Living Foundation, and on social welfare issues.

Index

Items are arranged in order by *significant* words. References are to item numbers, except where page numbers are given. Periodical titles have capitalized initials. Frequently used abbreviations and acronyms are included.